The
Early Stages of
Schizophrenia

Edited by

Robert B. Zipursky, M.D.

S. Charles Schulz, M.D.

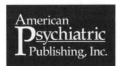

American
Psychiatric
Publishing, Inc.

Washington, DC
London, England

Note: The authors have worked to ensure that all information in this book concerning drug dosages, schedules, and routes of administration is accurate as of the time of publication and consistent with standards set by the U.S. Food and Drug Administration and the general medical community. As medical research and practice advance, however, therapeutic standards may change. For this reason and because human and mechanical errors sometimes occur, we recommend that readers follow the advice of a physician who is directly involved in their care or the care of a member of their family. A product's current package insert should be consulted for full prescribing and safety information.

Books published by American Psychiatric Publishing, Inc., represent the views and opinions of the individual authors and do not necessarily represent the policies and opinions of APPI or the American Psychiatric Association.

Copyright © 2002 American Psychiatric Publishing, Inc.
ALL RIGHTS RESERVED

Manufactured in the United States of America on acid-free paper
05   04   03   02   01   5   4   3   2   1
First Edition

American Psychiatric Publishing, Inc.
1400 K Street, N.W.
Washington, DC 20005
www.appi.org

WM
203
E27
2001

Library of Congress Cataloging-in-Publication Data

The early stages of schizophrenia / edited by Robert B. Zipursky, S. Charles Schulz.
        p. cm.
    Includes bibliographical references and index.
    ISBN 0-88048-840-9 (alk. paper)
    1.Schizophrenia--Diagnosis. 2. Schizophrenia--Treatment. I. Zipursky, Robert B. II. Schulz, S. Charles.

RC514 .E25 2001
616.89'82--dc21

                                        2001034343

British Library Cataloguing in Publication Data
A CIP record is available from the British Library.

The
Early Stages of
Schizophrenia

Contents

Robert B. Zipursky, M.D.

S. Charles Schulz, M.D.

PART I

Early Intervention, Epidemiology, and Natural History of Schizophrenia

Patrick D. McGorry, M.D., Ph.D.

Alison R. Yung, M.B., M.P.M.

Lisa J. Phillips, B.Sc., M.Psych.

Evelyn J. Bromet, Ph.D.

Ramin Mojtabai, M.D., Ph.D.

Shmuel Fennig, M.D.

Jeffrey A. Lieberman, M.D.

PART II

Management of the Early Stages of Schizophrenia

PART III

Neurobiological Investigations of the
Early Stages of Schizophrenia

Contributors

Evelyn J. Bromet, Ph.D.
Professor of Psychiatry, State University of New York at Stony Brook, Stony Brook, New York

April A. Collins, M.S.W.
Manager, Schizophrenia and Continuing Care Program, Centre for Addiction and Mental Health, Toronto, Ontario, Canada

Marilyn A. Davies, Ph.D.
Assistant Professor, Department of Psychiatry, Case Western Reserve University School of Medicine and University Hospitals of Cleveland, Cleveland, Ohio

Shmuel Fennig, M.D.
Director of Outpatient Services, Shelvata Hospital, Tel Aviv, Israel

Robert L. Findling, M.D.
Associate Professor, Department of Psychiatry, Case Western Reserve University School of Medicine and University Hospitals of Cleveland, Cleveland, Ohio

Lee Friedman, Ph.D.
Assistant Professor, Department of Psychiatry, Case Western Reserve University School of Medicine, Cleveland, Ohio

John T. Kenny, Ph.D.
Clinical Assistant Professor, Department of Psychiatry, Case Western Reserve University; and Department of Psychology, Louis B. Stokes Department of Veterans Affairs Medical Center, Cleveland, Ohio

Sanjiv Kumra, M.D.
Assistant Professor, Department of Psychiatry, Albert Einstein College of Medicine and North Shore–Long Island Jewish Medical Center–Hillside Hospital, Glen Oaks, New York

Jeffrey A. Lieberman, M.D.
Professor and Vice-Chair of Psychiatry, Pharmacology, and Radiology, University of North Carolina School of Medicine, Chapel Hill, North Carolina

Elizabeth McCay, R.N., Ph.D.
Associate Professor, School of Nursing, Ryerson Polytechnic University; Assistant Professor, Department of Psychiatry and Faculty of Nursing, University of Toronto, Toronto, Ontario, Canada

Patrick D. McGorry, M.D., Ph.D.
Professor, Department of Psychiatry, The University of Melbourne; Director, Early Psychosis Prevention and Intervention Centre (EPPIC), Parkville, Victoria, Australia

Ramin Mojtabai, M.D., Ph.D.
Assistant Professor of Psychiatry, Columbia University, New York, New York

Robert Nicolson, M.D.
Assistant Professor, Department of Psychiatry, University of Western Ontario, London, Ontario, Canada

Lisa J. Phillips, B.Sc., M.Psych.
Research Fellow and Clinical Coordinator, Personal Assessment and Crisis Evaluation (PACE) Clinic, Youth Program, Parkville, Victoria, Australia

Judith L. Rapoport, M.D.
Chief, Child Psychiatry Branch, National Institute of Mental Health, Bethesda, Maryland

Kathryn Ryan, R.N., M.Sc.(N.)
Clinical Associate, Faculty of Nursing, University of Toronto; Advanced Practice Nurse, Schizophrenia and Continuing Care Program, Centre for Addiction and Mental Health, Toronto, Ontario, Canada

S. Charles Schulz, M.D.
Professor and Head, Department of Psychiatry, University of Minnesota Medical School, Minneapolis, Minnesota

Alison R. Yung, M.B., M.P.M.
Medical Director, Personal Assessment and Crisis Evaluation (PACE) Clinic, Youth Program, Parkville, Victoria, Australia

Robert B. Zipursky, M.D.
Professor and Tapscott Chair in Schizophrenia Studies, Department of Psychiatry, University of Toronto; Clinical Director, Schizophrenia and Continuing Care Program, Centre for Addiction and Mental Health, Toronto, Ontario, Canada

Introduction

Robert B. Zipursky, M.D.
S. Charles Schulz, M.D.

Our understanding of schizophrenia has changed dramatically over the past few decades. The introduction of atypical antipsychotic medications, shifts in social policy, and new research findings have had a profound impact on current thinking about the expected clinical outcomes of schizophrenia. Up until the late 1950s, patients with schizophrenia could be expected to spend much of their adult lives institutionalized. A very large majority of people with schizophrenia can now expect to live their lives in their communities. Research programs were developed in the 1980s to study patients at the beginning of their illness in order to characterize the factors that determine clinical outcome in schizophrenia. What has become clear is that a very high percentage of patients receiving treatment for their first episode of schizophrenia will achieve a full remission of symptoms, with many returning to very good levels of functioning. These findings have renewed hope that early intervention may have the potential to dramatically improve the long-term outcome of schizophrenia. Yet despite these reasons for optimism, early recognition of psychosis and a full, coordinated approach to treatment have not been the norm. It is the purpose of this book to assemble for the first time these new studies on the early stages of schizophrenia and to describe the clinical approaches likely to facilitate the fullest degree of recovery.

The realization that many patients will make a dramatic recovery from their first episode of schizophrenia has resulted in a remarkable shift in thinking about the goals of treatment. Over the past three decades, these goals have shifted from deinstitutionalization and stabilization in the community to remission of all psychotic symptoms. It is clear that our goal for the future must be to achieve the greatest possible functional recovery for all patients. This shift can, in part, be attributed to the impact of the reintroduction of clozapine to North America in the late 1980s. Up until that time, all antipsychotic medications were considered to be of equal efficacy, differing only in the relative intensity of side effects. The multicenter North American clozapine trial established that many treatment-resistant patients can experience improvement from a different medication, that improvement can occur in many domains independent of improvement in positive symptoms, and that incremental improvement in some domains can result in dramatic improvements in functional ability and quality of life. The introduction of the new generation of antipsychotic medications (i.e., the atypical antipsychotic agents) can be expected to have a profound impact on the treatment of patients with schizophrenia. Not only will we be able to enhance the response of those who have responded poorly to treatment in the past, but we can also expect to achieve response with a minimum of side effects. The greater tolerability of the new medications may, in turn, dramatically shift the balance of risks and benefits involved in intervening with individuals in the early stages of the illness.

With this surge of interest in early intervention, several fundamental questions have arisen about the determinants of outcome. What distinguishes those who recover from those who do not? Are there neuroanatomical, neurochemical, electrophysiological, cognitive, or syndromal differences that account for the variance in outcome? To what extent can these factors be modulated by treatment? Why is the long-term outcome of schizophrenia less positive than the outcome from the first episode? Although it had become customary to categorize long-term outcome from schizophrenia as "good" or "poor," this dichotomous approach is no longer viable. It is now appreciated that outcome must be conceptualized as being of greater complexity and must include levels of symptomatology, life satisfaction, and measures of functioning across a broad range of domains. It has also become very clear that the clinical needs of patients in the early stages of schizophrenia are very different from those of patients who have been chronically ill. These differences need to be reflected in the inpatient and outpatient services provided to these individuals and in the treatment modalities used, be they antipsychotic medication, psychotherapy, family intervention, or psychosocial rehabilitation.

Despite these changes, most clinical services for schizophrenia today are geared toward those who have been chronically ill, with a paucity of services generally available that are directed at the needs of those in the early stages of the illness. This is not the usual model applied to other chronic medical illnesses such as diabetes. Would it not be reasonable to provide services that meet the specialized needs of patients early in their course of illness so that long-term disability may be prevented and patients are provided the best chance of achieving an excellent long-term outcome? This book was written to address this question and to describe the issues that must be understood to help these patients and their families.

To fully understand the issues involved in the early stages of schizophrenia, it is necessary to be familiar with what schizophrenia looks like early in its course and what the spectrum of outcomes is likely to be. The first section of this book, "Early Intervention, Epidemiology, and Natural History" provides this background.

Chapter 1, "'Closing In': What Features Predict the Onset of First-Episode Psychosis Within an Ultra-High-Risk Group?" by Patrick McGorry, Alison Yung, and Lisa Phillips, describes the authors' innovative work in characterizing the prodromal phase of schizophrenia and conceptualizing models for treatment at this stage. Schizophrenia is rarely an illness of acute onset; rather, most patients experience a prodromal phase of increasing social isolation, deterioration in functioning, and slowly evolving psychotic symptoms that may last for many months and, more often, years. There is very frequently a prolonged delay between the onset of psychotic symptoms and treatment. McGorry and his colleagues in Melbourne, Australia, have had an enormous impact in increasing our understanding of this phase of the illness and in initiating discussion about the possibility of intervening at this point. What has been unique about their contribution has been the focus on those individuals who appear to be on the very cusp of becoming psychotic. In the past, discussion of intervening with individuals at risk has been stifled by concerns about the low specificity of predictive factors and the risk of identifying false-positive cases. Recognizing that many patients who go on to develop schizophrenia are highly symptomatic in the months and years before they become acutely psychotic and often seek treatment for these symptoms, Dr. McGorry and colleagues have catalyzed a rapidly growing international effort to develop effective early intervention strategies to prevent the onset of psychosis.

Chapter 2, by Evelyn Bromet, Ramin Mojtabai, and Shmuel Fennig, describes "Epidemiology of First-Episode Schizophrenia: The Suffolk

County Mental Health Project," a study of first-episode psychosis. The fundamental issue that this study addresses is: "What is the long-term outcome after a first episode of psychosis?" The answer to this question has eluded psychiatrists throughout the past century. Even to this day, it is difficult to know what the long-term outcome from schizophrenia really looks like. As Dr. Bromet and her coauthors make clear in this chapter, much of the uncertainty can be traced to variability in study designs. Epidemiological studies that involve an unbiased cohort of patients at the beginning of psychotic illness are ideal for understanding the long-term course of schizophrenia. For the past 10 years, Dr. Bromet and her colleagues have been conducting such a study on Long Island, New York. Their study provides invaluable knowledge about the distribution of psychiatric diagnoses among patients with a first episode of psychosis, the stability of these diagnoses over time, and the outcome from these diagnoses over time.

Chapter 3, "Investigating the Early Stages of Schizophrenia: The Hillside Prospective Study of First-Episode Schizophrenia" by Jeffrey Lieberman, summarizes the results of the monumental research in this area conducted by Dr. Lieberman and his colleagues at the Hillside Hospital on Long Island, New York, beginning in 1986. The results from this study have had enormous impact on our understanding of schizophrenia and its treatment and provide the foundation for much of the current clinical and research work in this field. Many of the findings in this study have profound implications for the treatment of first-episode patients: the long duration of untreated psychosis, the large percentage of patients who achieve a full remission in symptoms, the diminished treatment response in subsequent episodes, the very high rates of relapse in the first 5 years of follow-up, and the linear increase in the risk of tardive dyskinesia beginning in the first years of treatment. These finding have had—and will continue to have—enormous impact on our thinking about early intervention, maintenance treatment, and optimal pharmacologic management of first-episode patients.

The second section of this book, "Management of the Early Stages of Schizophrenia," provides an overview of treatment strategies for helping patients experiencing their first episode of psychosis. To work effectively in this field, clinical care needs to take place in the context of a clear understanding of how this illness affects patients and their families.

Chapter 4, by Robert Zipursky, discusses the "Optimal Pharmacologic Management of the First Episode of Schizophrenia." This chapter draws heavily on the clinical experience that Dr. Zipursky and his colleagues have accumulated over the past 8 years in the First Episode Psychosis Program at the University of Toronto. The pharmacologic management of patients with a first episode of schizophrenia must go beyond discussion of "what drug in what amount?" A framework for the optimal use of antipsychotic medications is provided. Dr. Zipursky and his colleagues have demonstrated that many patients in their first episode of psychosis respond very well to relatively small doses of typical and atypical antipsychotic agents. The impact of these findings have been greatly strengthened by the demonstration that these small doses lead to substantial levels of dopamine D_2 receptor occupancy, as demonstrated in patients using positron emission tomography. What this means clinically is that it is now possible—and should, indeed, be expected—that first-episode patients can be effectively treated with few, if any, medication side effects. This represents a dramatic change in clinical practice over the past decade. Determining which medications will lead to the fullest degree of recovery remains a challenge for future research.

Chapter 5, by Elizabeth McCay and Kathryn Ryan, provides an introduction to the topic of "Meeting the Patient's Emotional Needs." Schizophrenia remains among the most poorly understood and highly stigmatized of all illnesses. The process by which patients adapt to becoming ill with schizophrenia is critically important to understand. We expect a great deal from these young patients whose grip on reality has been disturbed. We expect them to accept a medical diagnosis, accept medications, and comply with our recommendations in the long term. It is imperative that we understand the experience of our patients so we can find ways to engage them in both the acute and the ongoing treatment required to give them the best chance of recovery. Although the complex symptoms of schizophrenia contribute directly to the limitations in functioning that many patients experience, it is equally clear that poor psychological and emotional adjustment to having schizophrenia can affect the patient's long-term level of functioning and quality of life. Being diagnosed with schizophrenia may have a devastating impact on the person's sense of self. The authors describe the process of "illness engulfment" that results when patients' self-concept is increasingly organized around the illness and the patient role. Strategies for minimizing the trauma of becoming psychotic and the process of illness engulfment are described based on the authors' review of the literature as well as their research findings and their extensive clinical experience.

Chapter 6, by April Collins, reviews the literature on "Family Intervention in the Early Stages of Schizophrenia." Because most patients are

in their teenage or early adult years when they become ill with schizophrenia, they are usually still very closely involved with their families.
This means that engaging the patient in treatment almost always involves
engaging the family as well. Furthermore, efforts to assist patients in coping with their illness need to be complemented by efforts to support the
families in which they function. As April Collins makes clear in her historical overview, family involvement in the treatment of patients with
schizophrenia has most recently focused on strategies for minimizing relapse through intervening with families with high expressed emotion.
Family education programs, developed in part to neutralize this effect,
are by now well-established modalities of treatment in the management
of schizophrenia. It is critically important that we not overlook the subjective experience of family members. Coping with an adult child who
has become psychotic, who has been diagnosed with schizophrenia, and
who faces an uncertain future that may involve a high level of disability
represents a challenge of unfathomable proportion. The issues and challenges facing the parents of a young person just diagnosed with schizophrenia are often quite distinct from the issues parents face when the
illness has persisted for many years. Family support groups that have
been developed for the support of families coping with chronic schizophrenia may be inappropriate for many families coping with a first episode, because these families have very special needs. They need to be
actively and rapidly engaged with the treatment team to facilitate the recovery process. They also need our attention to ease their pain and suffering and to allow them to adapt to the challenges of having a child or
sibling with schizophrenia.

The third section of the book focuses on "Neurobiological Investigations of the Early Stages of Schizophrenia." Much of the interest in early
intervention in schizophrenia is focused on treating patients early in their
course of illness. In parallel with this, there has been a great deal of interest in another form of early intervention—intervention with those who
are developing signs of schizophrenia early in life, that is, as children and
adolescents. Many issues arise in considering patients in this age group
who have signs of schizophrenia. Are childhood- and adolescent-onset
schizophrenia continuous with the adult form of the disorder? If a similar
pathophysiology is being expressed, will the impact be different in terms
of both brain structure and function when younger individuals are affected? Adolescents and children are likely to require different clinical approaches both for pharmacologic and psychosocial interventions than
adults with a first episode.

Chapter 7, "Childhood-Onset Schizophrenia: Research Update" by Sanjiv Kumra, Robert Nicolson, and Judith Rapoport describes research that has been carried out at the National Institute of Mental Health on children with schizophrenia. Although childhood-onset schizophrenia is an extremely rare disorder, understanding the factors that contribute to very early onset forms of the illness may provide insights into the neurobiology of schizophrenia. Dr. Rapaport and her associates have carried out extensive studies investigating the clinical, genetic, and morphological brain findings in a unique cohort of patients with childhood-onset schizophrenia. They make a strong case for considering the childhood-onset form of the disorder as a more severe variant of the adult-onset form. Few systematic data are available to guide the pharmacologic management of these children. Dr. Rapaport's group has carried out a number of remarkable treatment studies involving these children. These studies are reviewed and discussed in their chapter.

Chapter 8, by Charles Schulz, Robert Findling, and Marilyn Davies, focuses on the topic of "Schizophrenia During Adolescence." Although the onset of schizophrenia is relatively more common in the teenage years, there is a paucity of research involving this group. Dr. Schulz and colleagues focus their review on the epidemiology of adolescent-onset schizophrenia and studies of brain imaging and treatment response in this group. Although the biological findings are similar to those seen in adults, their work with magnetic resonance imaging bolsters a neurodevelopmental conceptualization of schizophrenia by demonstrating differences between patients and control subjects studied during this important stage of life. It is clearly important to think of adolescents with schizophrenia as a different group and not as smaller, younger adults with schizophrenia. They may differ in pharmacologic response, sensitivity to side effects, and the therapeutic approach needed.

Chapter 9, by John Kenny and Lee Friedman, reviews the literature on "Cognitive Impairment in Early-Stage Schizophrenia" and describes their research on cognition in adolescents with schizophrenia. In the past decade, we have witnessed a surge in research on cognition in schizophrenia. Two principal interests have motivated this work. First, understanding patterns of cognitive dysfunction in schizophrenia may inform us about the regional distribution of neural dysfunction in schizophrenia. Second, the disability associated with schizophrenia may be related to a substantial degree to the pattern and severity of cognitive dysfunction experienced. Characterizing this dysfunction is a necessary first step toward understanding how to help those affected improve these deficits or manage with them. It has been particularly important to determine when during the course of illness cognitive dysfunction becomes apparent. To what extent does it exist premorbidly and reflect an underlying vulnerability to developing schizophrenia? Alternatively, it could be that cognitive dysfunction develops during the prodrome or early in the course of the illness. If this is the case, are there interventions that could prevent or limit the cognitive deficits? Answering these questions is critical if we are to develop effective treatment strategies for patients in the early stages of schizophrenia.

It is hoped that the information provided in this book will help clinicians develop the interest and expertise necessary to work effectively with patients and families dealing with a first episode of schizophrenia. In the Afterword, we synthesize the information presented by describing a comprehensive, multidisciplinary approach to facilitating recovery in patients who have experienced a first episode of psychosis. This is an area with great clinical challenges. The potential to help those in need of this specialized expertise is enormous. The failure to meet these same needs can exact an equally large cost in terms of ongoing disability, risk of suicide, and family turmoil. As we embark on the new millennium, there is good cause to be optimistic that intervention early in the illness will improve the long-term outcome from schizophrenia for future generations.

PART I

Early Intervention, Epidemiology, and Natural History of Schizophrenia

"Closing In"

What Features Predict the Onset of First-Episode Psychosis Within an Ultra-High-Risk Group?

Patrick D. McGorry, M.D., Ph.D.

Alison R. Yung, M.B., M.P.M.

Lisa J. Phillips, B.Sc., M.Psych.

The accurate identification and treatment of people before the onset of frank psychotic symptoms in schizophrenia and related disorders has long been a goal of clinicians. To achieve this goal, a number of building blocks must be in place, the first of which is the capacity to predict those at very high risk of early transition to full-fledged psychotic disorder.

The authors gratefully acknowledge the major contribution of the following colleagues to the work described in this chapter: Hok Pan Yuen, Dennis Velakoulis, Shona Francey, Warrick Brewer, Nicholas Crump, Narelle Hearn, George C. Patton, Christos Pantelis, and Henry J. Jackson. The PACE clinical research program has received financial support from the Victorian Health Promotion Foundation, the National Health and Medical Research Council, the Stanley Foundation, the National Alliance for Research in Schizophrenia and Depression, and the Victorian State Government's Department of Human Services. We sincerely acknowledge the support of all these agencies.

Although psychopathological features alone are unlikely to be sufficiently powerful to distinguish perfectly between those who do and those who do not proceed to a first psychotic episode, it is probable that they can play an important part. Additional variables likely to play a part include historical variables (e.g., family history, perinatal birth complications, delayed developmental milestones, childhood behavioral patterns, and head injury) and probable trait variables (e.g., neurocognitive impairments and neurological "soft signs"). Using the strategy of sequential screening, combinations of relatively simplified state and trait risk factors for psychosis were used to operationally define a putatively high-risk group. The effect of these criteria was that all participants manifested some form of psycho-pathological disturbance at entry to the study, thus differentiating the research strategy from the traditional high-risk paradigm in which subjects are typically asymptomatic. The current strategy is, therefore, a form of "indicated prevention," in which subthreshold symptoms are targeted to reduce the risk of a full-fledged disorder. Operationalized "exit" criteria for the onset of psychosis were also established. Subjects were assessed monthly on measures of psychopathology for 12 months. Twenty of 49 patients made the transition to frank psychosis within the 12-month follow-up period, with most developing nonaffective psychoses. A range of analyses, including survival analysis, was used to examine the relationship of predictor variables from several domains to the risk of transition to psychosis. We have demonstrated that it is possible to identify individuals with ultra high risk (UHR) of onset of psychosis within a relatively brief follow-up period of 1 year. Mental state changes have modest predictive power on their own within such a sample. However, when combined with variables from other domains, we hypothesized that incipient psychosis could be predicted with increased accuracy. Although this was only true to a limited extent, these findings begin to lay a foundation for prepsychotic intervention that aims to prevent, delay, or minimize the severity of the first onset of psychotic disorders.

Introduction

The Prepsychotic Phase

Schizophrenia and other psychotic disorders are usually characterized by a prepsychotic, or "prodromal," phase of illness that involves a change from premorbid functioning and extends up to the time of onset of frank psychotic features (Beiser et al. 1993; Keith and Matthews 1991; Loebel et al. 1992). Several studies have demonstrated that this period may be lengthy, lasting on average between 2 and 5 years (Beiser et al. 1993; Häfner et al. 1993; Loebel et al. 1992), and is associated with substantial levels of psychosocial impairment and disability, even though, by definition, no frank positive psychotic symptoms have yet appeared (Häfner et al. 1995a, 1995b; Jones et al. 1993). Earlier recognition of this issue prompted several key authors to call for the treatment of individuals even before the onset of the first psychotic episode (Cameron 1938; Meares 1959; Sullivan 1927). Sullivan, as early as 1927, made the following statement:

> I feel certain that many incipient cases might be arrested before the efficient contact with reality is completely suspended, and a long stay in institutions made necessary. (Sullivan 1927, p. 105)

Even if the onset of psychosis could only be delayed, this might result in significant reductions in morbidity and a consequent decrease in both the human and economic costs of the disorder:

> the longer psychotic collapse is escaped, the less the chance of a grave disorder, and the less typical any illness which ensues. In other words a psychosis occurring in a psychopathic youth under, say, the age of 22, is in all likelihood frankly schizophrenic; but an initial psychosis occurring at, say, 30 will probably be a brief excitement. (Sullivan 1927, p. 112)

This opinion is partially supported by the fact that the outcome for adolescent patients with early-onset schizophrenia is significantly worse than that for patients with an onset in middle to late adult life (Krausz and Muller-Thomsen 1993). Even the deferment of psychosis by 1 year without any lessening of subsequent morbidity would dramatically reduce the costs of treating the patient with disorder (J.O. Johanssen, personal communication, October 24, 1998). For example, for treated incidence data limited to the age range of 16–30 years, if the direct costs of treating people with psychosis in their first year of illness are approximately AUS$17,000 (Mihalopolous et al. 1999), then the maximum level of potential savings annually for a developed country such as Australia with a population of 18 million would be approximately AUS$80 million. If the full age range (up to 45 or 65 years) is included, the savings would be significantly greater. These calculations are approximate and assume that all cases could be deferred by 1 year, but they give some idea of the scale of possible savings. However, they would be offset by the costs (much lower) of community-based preventive prepsychotic intervention.

It should be remembered that these calculations only include direct costs (i.e., the cost of providing specialist mental health services), so the magnitude of savings could be several times greater if indirect costs were included. If this calculation were carried out for the United States or the whole world (with costs derived from the cost of care in the relevant country), the impact of delaying onset would be very considerable indeed. If a proportion of cases could be prevented completely or their course ameliorated as well as delayed, further savings would clearly result. The reduction in human and social costs of the disorders would be correspondingly striking.

A Framework for Prevention

To achieve any ambitious goal of this kind, a plan is required. Fortunately, a blueprint for prevention in psychiatry in general has recently been produced, and it has special clarity in relation to the hitherto confusing and elusive notion of prepsychotic intervention (Mrazek and Haggerty 1994). When we were embarking on our early work in this area, we noted that many people were becoming confused by the notion of prodrome and its retrospective-only denotation. Some clinicians saw the symptoms not as at-risk mental states (ARMS) but rather as early signs (i.e., early pathognomonic features). This stemmed from the experience of thinking only from a perspective of first-episode psychosis and from a necessary and sufficient causal model, that of inevitable progression, as in Huntington's disease. What was needed was an epidemiological model based on risk factors and contributory causes. From such a standpoint, the issue of false-positives and even false-false-positives (i.e., nonprogression even though a state of substantial risk existed) can be better appreciated. The risks and benefits of intervention before the emergence of frank psychosis can then be more clearly considered. Mrazek and Haggerty's (1994) model of the spectrum of preventive interventions is an advance on the older primary, secondary, and tertiary prevention classification and can be summarized as follows.

Broadly, interventions can be classified into prevention, treatment, and maintenance. Within prevention, drawing on the ideas of Gordon (1983) and Mrazek and Haggerty (1994), we subclassify interventions as universal, selective, and indicated. Universal preventive interventions are targeted to the general public or a whole population group that has not been identified on the basis of individual risk (e.g., use of seat belts, immunization, prevention of smoking). Selective preventive measures are appropriate for subgroups of the population whose risk of becoming ill is above average. Examples include special immunizations, such as for people traveling to areas where yellow fever is endemic, and annual mammograms for women with a family history of breast cancer. The subjects are clearly asymptomatic. This has been the level of prevention underpinning the traditional high-risk studies in schizophrenia, including a recent modification of this paradigm, the Edinburgh High-Risk Study (Hodges et al. 1999). In contrast, indicated preventive measures apply to those individuals who on examination are found to manifest a risk factor that identifies them as being at high risk for the future development of a disease and, as such, could be the focus of screening. Gordon's view was that such individuals should be asymptomatic and "not motivated by current suffering," yet have a clinically demonstrable abnormality. An example would be asymptomatic individuals with hypertension. However, this definition is not sufficiently different in practical terms from selective prevention; therefore, Mrazek and Haggerty decided to adapt Gordon's concept as follows:

> Indicated preventive interventions for mental disorders are targeted to high-risk individuals who are identified as having minimal but detectable signs or symptoms foreshadowing mental disorder, or biological markers indicating predisposition for mental disorder, but who do not meet DSM-III-R diagnostic levels at the current time. (Mrazek and Haggerty 1994, p. 154)

This major definitional shift allows individuals with early or subthreshold features (and, therefore, a degree of suffering and disability) to be included within the focus of indicated prevention. Some clinicians, adhering to an inappropriately deterministic view of psychosis, regard this as early intervention or an early form of treatment; however, the situation with these individuals is not so clear cut. Although some of these patients clearly have an early form of the disorder in question, others do not. They may, however, have other less serious disorders, and most individuals who are subthreshold for a potentially serious disorder such as schizophrenia may have nevertheless crossed a clinical threshold past which they either require or request treatment. Eaton et al. (1995) warned that the absence of firm data on the validity of the classification system enjoins us to be careful about conceptualizing the process of disease onset. Parenthetically, many of the issues discussed here are relevant to defining caseness and thresholds for initiating treatment in a range of mental disorders (Mrazek and Haggerty 1994). In schizophrenia, the threshold has been set high and requires not only the presence of positive psychotic symptoms but also a 6-month duration of illness. This is because of a combination of historical factors, widespread therapeutic nihilism, and the social implications of the diagnosis. The height of the bar is set at a much lower level for other disorders (e.g., depression, in which these factors do not apply). The high threshold may have contributed to treatment delay (Loebel et al. 1992) and thus added to the risk of poor outcome because most of the psychosocial damage occurs during the pretreatment phase (Häfner et al. 1995a, 1995b; Jones et al. 1993). The essence of this paper is to question the clinical threshold for treating "psychosis spectrum disorders." Ultimately, however, although we might not agree with the threshold set by the DSM or ICD for receiving a diagnosis of a mental disorder such as schizophrenia, if this is the current criterion for caseness, then an intervention aimed at preventing the further evolution of symptoms such that the threshold is reached does strictly meet the definition of indicated prevention because it aims at reducing the occurrence of new cases. If we can successfully argue for interventions at this phase or level of symptoms and disability, then, by current convention, it should be regarded as indicated prevention and not (early) treatment per se, though this distinction may be of dubious relevance to the patient. The persisting ambiguities are discussed below.

Characterizing the Prodromal Phase

> We do need to learn all we can from the life history of the people who have had schizophrenic illnesses....We will get data which can gradually be refined into dependable criteria as to impending schizophrenia. (Sullivan as cited in Cameron 1938, p. 580)

Seventy years after Sullivan's comments, we still lack clear criteria for impending psychosis. The attempt in DSM-III-R (American Psychiatric Association 1987) to define such criteria was unsuccessful because it had neither an empirical nor a theoretical basis (Jackson et al. 1995).

Various research strategies have been used to define typical prodromal features in an attempt to develop better criteria to predict incipient psychosis. These have been reviewed in more detail previously (Yung and McGorry 1996).

Retrospective Reconstruction of the Prodrome

One method is the detailed retrospective reconstruction from patient and informant interviews of the changes from premorbid personality through the prodromal phase up to the onset of frank psychosis. The most methodologically sound studies are those of Häfner et al. (1992) in Mannheim, Germany, who developed a systematic assessment tool to map the onset of psychosis known as the Instrument for the Retrospective Assessment of the Onset of Schizophrenia (IRAOS). This group applied the IRAOS to a cohort of 133 subjects with schizophrenia (including 115 first-episode cases). They found that 73% of patients experienced a prodrome that lasted, on average, 5 years. This phase characteristically began with negative symptoms such as decreased concentration, reduced drive and anergia, nonspecific symptoms such as anxiety and irritability, and affective symptoms such as depressed mood. These symptoms accumulated exponentially, generally culminating in the late emergence of positive symptoms and a more florid initial psychotic episode. On average, social disability appeared 2–4 years before the first psychotic episode and contact with mental health services (Häfner et al. 1998).

Another study involved detailed unstructured and semistructured interviews of first-episode psychosis patients focusing on the prodromal phase of illness. Qualitative analysis revealed that the most common prodromal features were nonspecific symptoms such as sleep disturbance, anxiety, irritability, depressed mood, poor concentration and fatigue, and behaviors such as deterioration in role functioning and social withdrawal. Suspiciousness, an attenuated or subthreshold psychotic symptom, was also frequently reported (in more than 70% of the patients) (Yung and McGorry 1996).

Relapse Prodromes as a Model for Initial Prodrome

Limitations of this retrospective reconstruction design are recall bias, effort after meaning, and problems of recall if subjects are still psychotic at the time of interview. A different strategy for describing incipient psychosis is to use the relapse prodrome (the prodrome preceding a psychotic relapse) as a model for the prodrome preceding the first psychotic episode (the initial prodrome). This has been done prospectively by studying patients with diagnosed psychotic illnesses and recording features leading up to relapse. The problem with this method is that it has not been established how the signs and symptoms of a relapse prodrome in patients with schizophrenia relate to the prodromal features of a first psychotic episode. This is particularly so because some symptoms may be modified by such factors as medication, residual symptoms, the fear of relapse and hospitalization, and the family's changing perception of the patient. In addition, the issue of when treatment is reinstituted also arises.

Too early an increase or recommencement of medication could lead to the identification and treatment of "false-positive prodromes" (i.e., changes in mental state that would not have developed into psychotic relapse if left unmedicated). Reintroduction that is too late or an increase in treatment would, obviously, be unethical. Various studies (Birchwood 1992; Birchwood et al. 1989; Heinrichs and Carpenter 1985; Herz and Melville 1980; Subotnik and Nuechterlein 1988; Tarrier et al. 1991) have used this method. Using this strategy, nonspecific mood and anxiety symptoms are again frequently described, as well as attenuated forms of psychotic symptoms such as perceptual abnormalities and suspiciousness. The design can be applied to the initial psychotic prodrome, but the content needs to be modified for the above reasons.

Basic Symptoms Approach

The Bonn-Cologne group of Huber, Gross, and Klosterkötter have developed a stronger theoretical and empirical base for investigating psychotic prodromes and impending psychosis linked to the concept of "basic symptoms"—subjectively experienced neuropsychological deficits, particularly in the realms of cognition, attention, perception, and movement (Klosterkotter et al. 1996). These authors have examined the predictive capacity of these putatively specific prodromal symptoms using both retrospective (Huber et al. 1980) and prospective (Klosterkötter et al. 1997, 2001) designs. The retrospective study investigated the prodromal features of a large cohort ($n=502$) of patients with schizophrenia. Basic symptoms were found in the schizophrenic prodrome, with onset of prodromal basic symptoms occurring on average 3.3 years before onset of first psychotic episode (Huber et al. 1980). The prospective study assessed the presence of basic symptoms in a cohort of nonpsychotic patients attending a tertiary referral psychiatric setting. Presenting diagnoses were mainly mood, anxiety, and somatoform and personality disorders. Subjects were followed up for an average of approximately 10 years after initial assessment, and over this period approximately 50% of them had developed schizophrenia. Certain basic symptoms—cognitive, perceptual, and motor disturbances—were found significantly more often in the group that developed schizophrenia than in the group that did not, suggesting that these symptoms may be predictors of schizophrenia (Klosterkötter et al. 2001). Until recently, however, this work has not been clearly understood or accorded widespread attention in anglophone psychiatry.

In all, characteristic prodromal features include nonspecific symptoms such as anxiety; depressed mood; reduced drive, energy, and concentration; sleep disturbances; and behavioral changes such as deterioration in role functioning and attenuated forms of psychotic symptoms (e.g., perceptual abnormalities and suspiciousness) (Yung and McGorry 1996). The attenuated positive symptoms are generally late phenomena (Häfner et al. 1993). It is important to be aware that attenuated or isolated positive symptoms also occur in the general population and may be "nonclinically significant" (van Os et al. 2000) or may be a developmentally normative phenomenon (Verdoux et al. 1998). How, then, can this knowledge be applied to identify impending psychosis—that is, to detect individuals about to develop psychosis?

Identifying Prodromal Changes Prospectively: The Challenge of False Positives

Retrospective studies of prodromal symptoms and signs cannot lead to the development of predictive criteria because two cells of the 2 × 2 table are missing. Particularly critical is the group of people who manifested changes in psychopathology (termed by us an ARMS rather than a prodrome) (Yung et al. 1996) but failed to become psychotic (cell B in Figure 1–1).

It is likely that some individuals experienced prodrome-like symptoms but did not make the transition to psychosis—that is, they were false-positives. In fact, because of the nonspecific nature of many prodromal features (e.g., depressed mood, anxiety, low energy), most individuals experiencing them would not go on to develop a psychotic disorder. Hence, we cannot use the term *prodrome* prospectively because the term implies the inevitable progression to onset of psychosis. Cross-sectionally, this apparent prodrome is better termed an ARMS, suggesting that the person is at risk of developing a psychosis but that psychosis is not inevitable (McGorry and Singh 1995; McGorry et al. 1995).

	Became psychotic	Did not become psychotic
"At Risk Mental State"	a	b
No "At Risk Mental State"	c	d

Figure 1–1. 2 × 2 table for prediction of psychosis using clinical features.

However, if we turn to prospective methods for identifying incipient psychosis, a large population-based prospective study would be too costly and impractical as a single-phase effort given the low base rate of schizophrenia and other psychoses and the large excess of false-positives (McGorry et al. 1995; van Os et al. 2000; Verdoux et al. 1998). A natural alternative is found in a series of attempts to narrow the focus of investigation to groups that, for various reasons, are more prone to develop psychosis than the general population (Yung and Jackson 1999). The Bonn study (Klosterkötter et al. 1996) used an enriched sample of tertiary referred patients, most of whom had high levels of basic symptoms. They were regarded by the study's authors as being susceptible to schizophrenia on the basis of their psychopathology. A conceptually similar strategy is that of Allen et al. (1987), Chapman and Chapman (1987), and Chapman et al. (1994), who also attempted to identify hypothetically psychosis-prone individuals on the basis of psychopathology. These researchers theorized that psychotic-like symptoms (attenuated forms of psychotic symptoms) and isolated psychotic symptoms are precursors of frank psychosis. They hypothezised that, over time, individuals with high levels of these features will have increased risks of developing psychotic disorder or spectrum disorder compared with control patients.

The authors recruited and assessed college students using specially designed instruments and followed up with them 10–15 years later. To date, results have been tantalizing but have failed to yield a practical method of prediction in real world settings (Chapman et al. 1994). Furthermore, there is increasing evidence that a significant yet small proportion of the general population may manifest attenuated or isolated psychotic symptoms without necessarily experiencing distress, disability, or an immediate desire or need for clinical care (van Os et al. 2000; Verdoux et al. 1998). It remains to be seen whether, as suggested by Chapman and Chapman, some of these individuals progress to more clear-cut clinical syndromes and would benefit from or require clinical intervention.

A more traditional approach, which contrasts markedly in scope and efficiency with the prospective prodromal focus, is to study family members of patients with schizophrenia (Asarnow 1988; Erlenmeyer-Kimling et al. 1995; Johnstone et al. 2000; Mednick et al. 1987). Thus, a group with a presumably increased genetic risk is being identified, and additional risk factors that make the transition to a frank psychotic disorder more likely can be examined. This is known as the high-risk approach, and assessments usually begin when subjects are children, with follow-up continuing longitudinally over many years. The aim is to detect the development of psychotic disorder at some stage in the person's life span. Mednick et al. (1987) modified this strategy by focusing on adolescent offspring who were entering the age of peak risk, an approach that made the high-risk paradigm more practical. Their strategy has been modified further recently by Eve Johnstone and colleagues, who have been focusing on adolescents with multiple first-degree relatives with a psychotic disorder (Hodges et al. 1999; Johnstone et al. 2000; Lawrie et al. 1999). Using modern research techniques, including magnetic resonance imaging, this strategy aims to clarify the neurobiology of transition as well as the prediction of psychosis in this particular subgroup of cases (Lawrie et al. 1999). Researchers using this approach acknowledge that the transition rate to a psychotic disorder is not likely to be large and that results may not be generalizable beyond the genetically defined high-risk group (Asarnow 1988).

The "Close-in" Strategy

Our group set out to combine multiple strategies for identifying high-risk individuals, including modifications of the previously discussed approaches. We had one additional aim, however, which was to identify a group at high risk of transition to *psychosis within a brief follow-up period* (i.e., a group at risk of impending psychosis, in contrast to the previously mentioned longer-term approaches). This approach, termed the "close-in" strategy (Bell 1992), enabled frequent detailed psychopathological assessment of subjects to occur, as well as assessment of other potential predictors such as neuroimaging and neurocognitive variables, and made it possible to map the psychopathological process of becoming psychotic. Unlike the past literature, which retrospectively investigated the prodromal features found in a group of psychotic subjects and examined the sensitivity of particular symptoms and signs (Yung and McGorry 1996), our approach enables examination of the positive predictive power of certain features within a clinically defined sample. This is more akin to how clinicians think—that is, if a patient has certain clinical features, what is the likelihood that he or she will develop the disorder? The current study provides a rigorous test of the potency of this "clinical" risk factor approach by prospectively studying the subjects. Prospective assessments in the group that had onset of psychosis can be compared with the assessments in the false-positive group (which did not develop psychosis). A number of potential risk factors can be examined and their positive predictive power in predicting psychosis can be studied. With refinement, criteria for impending psychosis may be definable that have a reasonable degree of specificity and are, therefore, useful for clinicians confronted by young persons possibly at risk of psychosis. We should add that our definition of *psychosis* here is a relatively arbitrary clinical one that represents the operationally defined threshold at which we, as clinicians, would decide to commence antipsychotic medication.

In our project, which aims at the short-term prediction of frank psychosis in a high-risk group, two different strategies for identifying subjects were used. These are described in the following sections.

Strategy 1: "Specific State" Risk Factors for Psychosis

The first strategy was predominantly a "state" or symptomatic approach similar to that used by Chapman and colleagues (Allen et al. 1987; Chapman and Chapman 1980; Chapman and Chapman 1987). Subjects were recruited who displayed symptoms that seemed likely to be precursors to frank psychosis—attenuated or subthreshold psychotic features, isolated self-limiting psychotic symptoms, or both. We regarded these features as indicative of an ARMS in their own right (i.e., even in the absence of a family history of psychotic disorder). We divided these features into two groups; operationalized criteria are detailed below. More details on the conceptual basis underpinning these inclusion criteria are given in earlier papers by our group (Yung et al. 1998a, 1998b).

Attenuated Group

Attenuated psychotic symptoms are defined by the presence of at least one of the following symptoms as defined in DSM-IV (American Psychiatric Association 1994): ideas of reference, odd beliefs or magical thinking, perceptual disturbance, odd thinking and speech, paranoid ideation, and odd behavior or appearance or schizotypal personality disorder. The symptom should deviate significantly from normal, as defined by a score of 1 or 2 on the hallucinations item of the Brief Psychiatric Rating Scale (BPRS; Overall and Gorham 1962), 2–3 on the unusual thought content item, or 2–3 on the suspiciousness item, or it should be held with a reasonable degree of conviction as defined by a score of 2 on the Comprehensive Assessment of Symptoms and History (CASH) rating scale for delusions (Andreasen et al. 1992). The symptom should occur with a frequency of at least several times a week, and the change in mental state should have been present for at least 1 week.

Transient Psychotic Symptoms Group

A history of transient psychotic symptoms (i.e., brief limited intermittent psychotic symptoms [BLIPS]) is defined by the presence of at least one of the following symptoms: hallucinations as defined by a score of 3 or more on the hallucinations item of the BPRS; delusions as defined by a score of 4 or more on the unusual thought content item or the suspiciousness item of the BPRS or held with strong conviction as defined by a score of 3 or more on the CASH rating for delusions; or formal thought disorder as defined by a score of 4 or more on the conceptual disorganization item of the BPRS. The duration of each BLIPS must be less than 1 week before resolving spontaneously.

Strategy 2: "Trait Plus State" Risk Factors for Psychosis

The second strategy for identifying our short-term high-risk study group was a modification of the genetic high-risk research approaches previously described. The modification we made was to apply the "close-in" strategy (Bell 1992) to the genetic high-risk approach. This involved combining trait risk factors for psychotic disorders with state risk factors. We chose the trait risk factors of family history of a first-degree relative with a history of any psychotic disorder (Gottesman and Shields 1982) or the presence of the schizophrenia spectrum disorder of schizotypal personality disorder in the subject (Claridge 1987; Kety et al. 1975; Meehl 1989). Presence of one of these trait risk factors was combined with the presence of an ARMS, which, in this group, could be limited to nonspecific neurotic-type presentations such as anxiety and depressive syndromes. The ARMS needed to be of sufficient severity and duration to produce a marked psychosocial deterioration. This was intended to raise the bar sufficiently to ensure that the person did truly require clinical attention and to avoid the risk of inappropriately labeling relatives of people with serious mental illness. Thus, we defined a group of subjects with a presumably increased genetic risk plus some (even nonspecific) ARMS features. Operationalized criteria for this familial group were a combination of a first-degree relative with a history of any psychotic disorder as defined by DSM-IV or a schizotypal personality disorder as defined by DSM-IV and any change in mental state or functioning that resulted in a loss of 30 points or more on the Global Assessment of Functioning (GAF) scale (American Psychiatric Association 1994) for at least 1 month.

In addition, for all groups, the risk factor of age between 14 and 30 years—the period of maximum risk of becoming psychotic—was added.

Case Detection and Recruitment: Establishment of the PACE Clinic

To enhance our ability to recruit and follow up with a cohort of putatively UHR, or prodromal, subjects, a specialized community-based service for this group was established in 1994. The rationale for this was, first, that we needed to provide a clinical service for these young people. Existing mental health services in Australia almost exclusively serve patients with already-diagnosed psychotic illnesses (usually chronic schizophrenia) and, because of a limited health budget, individuals who do not meet diagnostic thresholds for such disorders are usually turned away. Second, we wanted to establish a low-stigma site so that the high-risk young people would not have to attend a psychiatric facility; although they might have a diagnosable mental disorder such as major depression, by definition they would not yet have a diagnosable psychotic disorder.

The service was named the Personal Assessment and Crisis Evaluation (PACE) Clinic and is located at the Centre for Adolescent Health, a generalist outpatient service and health promotion center for adolescents. Recently PACE has established clinical rooms within a large, suburban shopping center in Melbourne. Young people are offered a clinical service through a case management system and are given the opportunity to take part in research. The clinical component consists of dealing with patients' current difficulties and distress. This could include, for example, supportive psychotherapy, practical help and case management, drug and alcohol counseling, and treatment of symptoms such as depression and anxiety. Monitoring individuals for any sign of impending psychosis is another clinical component. Neuroleptic medication was not used until late 1996 and only then under carefully controlled circumstances as part of an exploratory research study of treatment alternatives for this group of patients. The nonspecific interventions are important because the young people attending the clinic have special concerns and needs and are often quite disabled by their symptoms. The studies of Jones et al. (1993) and Häfner et al. (1995a, 1995b) reflect this phenomenon, reporting evidence of significant psychosocial decline before the onset of first psychotic episode in patients with schizophrenia. Additionally, the monitoring of the young people enables the earliest possible specific intervention after psychosis has emerged, such as low-dose neuroleptic medication, and therefore minimizes the severity of and disruption caused by the full-fledged psychosis.

To recruit individuals to the PACE Clinic, it was necessary to liaise with potential referrers, particularly organizations and individuals who come into contact with large numbers of help-seeking young people. Links were established with general practitioners, school and university student counseling services, youth workers, and community health and psychiatric clinics. Education about ARMS was given to these groups. A willingness to directly assess large numbers of potentially appropriate referrals also helped to detect cases because specialist referral options for young people with even serious problems are few in the Australian context. Additionally, young people were assessed both at the clinic and at their own homes, schools, or other sites convenient to them (Yung et al. 1996).

Thus, the PACE Clinic has a dual clinical and research focus; however, the clinical focus is ensured for all who are willing to attend, whether or not they participate in any research studies. A series of projects that have taken place in the clinic are briefly reviewed here.

The PACE Pilot Study

The first study (January 1994 to March 1995) aimed to establish whether it was possible to recruit high-risk "prodromal" patients and follow up with them over time. We also needed to determine the number of patients developing full-blown psychosis over the 1–2-year follow-up period to determine if our intake criteria required modification. For more details on the pilot intake criteria, see an earlier paper (Yung et al. 1996).

A total of 21 young people were recruited into the pilot research. Eighteen subjects were seen for 2-year follow-up, seven (33% of the original sample) of whom had become psychotic over the 2-year period despite receiving good psychosocial care. It should be emphasized that those who remained nonpsychotic may have been helped to do so by the nonspecific intervention and not all are necessarily false-positives. We coined the term *false-false-positives* for this scenario.

This first-wave study showed that it was possible to find high-risk young people and engage them with the clinic. It also led to the modification of our intake criteria, which were changed by eliminating the trait criterion of schizoid personality traits (from the trait plus state criteria) and allowing only first-degree relatives as a trait criterion (eliminating a history of psychosis in second-degree relatives as a criterion). Our experience in this initial phase also laid the groundwork for treatment approaches for these individuals. In addition, it highlighted the need for more clinical staff and more assertive education of potential referrers. Recruitment of cases also needs to be more assertive.

The PACE Prediction Study

The PACE Prediction Study started in March 1995 using the modified criteria detailed previously.

Aims

The aim of the project was to recruit a group of subjects with a high likelihood of transition to psychosis within a 12-month follow-up period and to assess degree of risk (percentage of high-risk patients actually developing psychosis), timing of onset, and mode of onset of psychosis by prospective follow-up of the sample. A further aim was to compare the group that became psychotic with the group that did not become psychotic to examine the predictive power of certain variables, including psychopathological, neurobiological, neurocognitive, and developmental markers.

Hypotheses

It was hypothesized that the rate of transition to psychosis over 12 months would be 30%–40% of cases. This estimate was based on our experience during the pilot study. However, the pilot study inclusion criteria were modified as described for this project in an attempt to increase the proportion of cases developing a psychosis. The reader is referred to a previous paper (Yung et al. 1996) for a more detailed discussion of the pilot data.

It was also hypothesized that subjects who became psychotic would manifest higher levels of psychopathology, neurobiological abnormalities, neurocognitive deficits, and developmental deviance than those who did not become psychotic in the follow-up period.

Sample

The sample was recruited from the northern and western regions (population, approximately 1 million) of metropolitan Melbourne, a city of approximately 3.5 million people in the southeast of Australia. Inclusion criteria were detailed previously. Exclusion criteria were intellectual disability, lack of fluency in English, presence of known organic brain disorder, and history of previous psychotic disorder for longer than 1 week (treated or untreated).

Instruments

Subjects were assessed at intake for the following:

1. Psychopathology, disability, and functioning

   - The BPRS (Overall and Gorham 1962) was used to assess positive symptoms. A modified version of 24 items rated on a 7-point scale with clearly defined anchor points was used (Lukoff et al. 1986). However, in line with other studies by our group, items were rated as 0–6 rather than 1–7.
   - The Scale for the Assessment of Negative Symptoms (SANS; Andreasen 1982) was used to assess negative symptoms.
   - The Hamilton Rating Scale for Depression (HRSD; Hamilton 1960), Hamilton Rating Scale for Anxiety (HRSA; Hamilton 1959), and Mania Rating Scale (Young et al. 1978) were used to assess depressive, anxiety, and manic features, respectively.
   - The Quality of Life Scale (QLS; Heinrichs et al. 1984) and the GAF (American Psychiatric Association 1994) were used to assess functioning and disability.
   - The drug and alcohol section of the Schedule for Clinical Assessment in Neuropsychiatry (SCAN; Wing et al. 1990) was used to assess substance use.

2. Brain structure

   - Magnetic resonance imaging brain scans using thin (1.5-mm) slices were done to measure brain structure and volume.

3. Neurocognitive functioning

   - The National Adult Reading Test (NART; Nelson and Willison 1991) was used to estimate premorbid intelligence.
   - The Controlled Oral Word Association Test (COWAT, Verbal Fluency Test; Benton and Hamsher 1983), Wisconsin Card Sorting Test (Heaton et al. 1993), and Trail Making Test (Army Individual Test Battery 1944) were used to assess executive functioning.
   - The Rey Auditory Verbal Learning Test (RAVLT; Lezak 1995) and Digit Symbol-Delay (from the Wechsler Memory Scale; Wechsler 1987) were used to assess memory.

4. Developmental history

   - The Family Interview for Genetic Studies (FIGS; Maxwell unpublished) was used to document family history of psychotic disorders.
   - The Lewis Obstetric Complications Scale (Lewis et al. 1989) was used to assess obstetric complications.
   - The Premorbid Adjustment Scale (PAS; Cannon-Spoor et al. 1982) was used to assess accomplishment of developmental goals.

- The schizoid and schizotypal traits items from the Personality Disorders Examination (PDE; Loranger 1988) were used to assess these personality aspects.
- Data were also collected on maternal age, general maternal history, and achievement of milestones such as walking and talking.

At monthly intervals, measures of psychopathology were repeated to monitor the development of psychotic features. An assessment was also made every month to record interventions that the person had received. A full Structured Clinical Interview for DSM-IV (SCID; First et al. 1996) was conducted with subjects after the development of psychosis to determine the DSM-IV diagnosis. Subjects who did not become psychotic had a SCID completed at 12-month follow-up to detect any other psychiatric disorders. The GAF and QLS were also repeated at the end of 12 months.

Results

Referrals

Between March 1995 and October 1996, 162 referrals were made to the PACE Clinic. Telephone screening assessment of these referrals excluded 23 (14.2%); the remaining 139 (85.8%) were offered a screening interview. Of those accepted, 44 never attended the appointment; the reasons for this are unknown. The other 95 (58.6% of the 162 referred) were seen in the clinic for direct assessment. Of these, 60 met the intake criteria and 35 did not. A total of 45 of these eligible young people consented to involvement in the research project. Reasons for not being recruited included refusal to participate ($n=13$) and being subsequently treated with neuroleptic medication by another (external) clinician (despite not being psychotic) ($n=2$). Additionally, four subjects were recruited into the study from the PACE Clinic itself. They were part of the previous (pilot) cohort and still met inclusion criteria at the time of completion of this project (March 1995). Thus, the total number in the research sample was 49.

Intake Criteria

Most subjects met the attenuated intake criterion ($n=35$). Twelve patients met the BLIPS criterion, and 18 patients met the trait marker criterion. There was a considerable degree of overlap between the groups. Six patients fulfilled both the trait criterion and the attenuated criterion, four subjects met both attenuated and BLIPS criteria, and two met both the trait and BLIPS criteria. Two subjects fulfilled all three criteria. Figure 1–2 illustrates this.

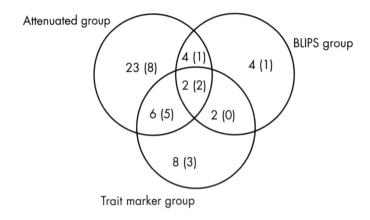

Attenuated group

BLIPS group

23 (8) 4 (1) 4 (1)

2 (2)

6 (5) 2 (0)

8 (3)

Trait marker group

Figure 1–2. Intake criteria, number, and number with transition to psychosis in parentheses. BLIPS = brief limited intermittent psychotic symptoms.

Transition to Psychosis

The main outcome measure in this study was the development of psychosis. We have discussed the difficulties in defining onset of a frank psychosis prospectively in a previous paper (Yung et al. 1996) and noted that this onset point needs to be arbitrarily defined. The BPRS was used to define a cut-off point at which psychosis is said to have begun. The operationalized criteria were:

A. Presence of at least one of the following symptoms:
   - Hallucinations as defined by a score of 3 or more on the hallucinations scale of the BPRS (Overall and Gorham 1962)
   - Delusions as defined by a score of 4 or more on the unusual thought content or suspiciousness scale of the BPRS or held with strong conviction as defined by a score of 3 or more on the CASH rating scale for delusions (Andreasen et al. 1992)
   - Formal thought disorder as defined by a score of 4 or more on the conceptual disorganization scale of the BPRS

B. Frequency of symptoms at least several times a week.
C. Duration of mental state change longer than 1 week.

This is similar to the definition of Larsen et al. (1996) and is in line with common clinical practice of when a decision would be made to commence neuroleptic treatment.

Over the 12-month follow-up period, 20 subjects became psychotic; therefore, the transition rate is 40.8% (20 of 49). Additionally, we have become aware of two other patients who have developed psychosis after 12 months, at 15 and 25 months, respectively. However, the whole sample has not yet been followed up over a longer period, and there may be other patients who developed psychosis after the 12-month point.

Diagnostically, 12 patients had an onset of a schizophrenia-like psychosis (11 schizophreniform and 1 schizophrenia), and 3 patients had affective psychoses (1 bipolar disorder and 2 major depression with psychotic features). One patient developed schizoaffective disorder (depressed type), and another had a brief psychosis with duration greater than 1 week. Two patients had psychotic disorder not otherwise specified, and diagnostic data is missing for one subject who became psychotic within 12 months.

Prediction of Psychosis

The predictive power of numerous variables was assessed using the chi-square test, *t* test or survival analysis, and Cox regression. Age and gender were not found to be significantly related to the onset of psychosis.

Neurobiological Variables. The ratios of left hippocampal volume to whole brain volume were significantly higher in the subgroup that progressed to psychosis compared with the subgroup that did not (Table 1–1). Importantly, this was because of a reduction in volume compared with normal control subjects in the subgroup that did not become psychotic, rather than an increase in volume in the subgroup who did. The latter, therefore, manifested normal hippocampal volumes (Phillips et al., under review).

Neurocognitive Variables. No neurocognitive variables tested were significantly predictive of psychosis onset in our sample.

Developmental Variables. Despite previous literature (Jones et al. 1994), retrospective assessment of obstetric complications, developmental milestones, childhood behaviors, and PAS score were not significantly associated with the development of psychosis. The only developmental variable linked to the subgroup that developed psychosis was maternal age. Both the mean (29.00 years compared with 25.75 years) and median (30.0 years compared with 25.0 years) maternal ages were higher in the psychotic group. The difference between the means was significant (*t* test, *P*=0.040).

Table 1–1. Comparison of hippocampal volumes between ultra-high-risk (UHR)–psychotic and –nonpsychotic patients (whole brain volume as covariant)

	Normal	UHR psychotic ($n=20$), mean (sd)	UHR non-psychotic ($n=40$), mean (sd)	Analysis of covariance, P value
Left hippocampus (mm³)	3050.9 (374.4)	2894.9 (309.1)	2615.1 (401.6)	F(2195)=20.41 P<0.0001
Right hippocampus (mm³)	3222.6 (402.03)	3047.1 (308.5)	2897.1 (458.8)	F(2195)=8.414 P<0.0001

Psychopathological, Illness, and Disability Variables. Figure 1–2 shows the number of subjects who met each inclusion criterion, with the number in each group who became psychotic within 12 months in brackets. Among the subjects who met only one criterion, 25% (1 of 4) of the BLIPS groups developed psychosis compared with 34.8% (8 of 23) of the attenuated group and 37.5% (3 of 8) of the trait marker group. Subjects who met both attenuated and trait criteria had a transition rate of 83.3% (5 of 6). However, membership of the BLIPS group, in addition to another criterion, added little to the risk (trait plus BLIPS, 0 of 2 [0%] and attenuated plus BLIPS, 1 of 4 [25%]). Both subjects who met all three criteria (100%) developed psychosis.

The time between the onset of symptoms and first contact with the PACE Clinic was significantly longer in the group that became psychotic (mean=915 days, SD=1,134) compared with the group that did not (mean=324 days, SD=347) (t test, P=0.035). The association was even more significant using survival analysis and Cox regression that used information on all 22 psychotic patients (P=0.0043).

The level of functioning, as assessed by the GAF, was significantly lower in the group that became psychotic (mean=52.7, SD=14.2) compared with the group that did not (mean=61.8, SD=13.5) (t test, P=0.029; Cox regression, P=0.0051).

For the analysis of repeated measures such as the BPRS and SANS scores, we needed to assume that these scores remained constant over a certain period of time. Because there were a number of subjects missing one or more monthly assessments, this period had to be longer than 30 days to avoid the loss of important information. The period chosen was 130 days (a forthcoming paper by Yung et al. [under review] has more details about this analysis).

Table 1–2 shows the *P* values associated with total BPRS score, BPRS psychotic subscales (i.e., unusual thought content, suspiciousness, hallucinations, conceptual disorganization), total SANS score, SANS subscales, HRSD, HRSA, and mania scale scores using Cox regression. Scores on BPRS total, BPRS psychotic subscales, SANS attention subscale, and HRSD were consistently highly significant.

The consistently highly significant predictors ($P < 0.01$ based on Cox regression) of time between the onset of symptoms and first contact with psychiatric services (duration)—GAF score, BPRS total, BPRS psychotic subscale score, SANS attention, and HRSD scores—were then dichotomized into a high-risk score and a low-risk score by establishing the point that gave the lowest *P* value using Cox regression. Using this method, the following high-risk scores were found: duration greater than 900 days, GAF score less than 51, BPRS total greater than 15, BPRS psychotic subscales score greater than 2, SANS attention score greater than 1, and HRSD score greater than 18.

Table 1–2. Results of Cox regression (*P* values)

Scales	*P*
Brief Psychiatric Rating Scale—total	0.00024
Brief Psychiatric Rating Scale—psychotic subscales	0.00022
Scale for the Assessment of Negative Symptoms—total	0.10000
Scale for the Assessment of Negative Symptoms— affective flattening	0.49000
Scale for the Assessment of Negative Symptoms—alogia	0.55000
Scale for the Assessment of Negative Symptoms— avolition-apathy	0.04000
Scale for the Assessment of Negative Symptoms— anhedonia-asociality	0.05900
Scale for the Assessment of Negative Symptoms—attention	0.00064
Hamilton Rating Scale for Depression	0.00016
Hamilton Rating Scale for Anxiety	0.00910

Substance Use.   Only cannabis use was examined in the sample. Cannabis dependence, as defined by the SCID (American Psychiatric Association 1994), at intake was significantly associated with subsequent development of psychosis. The data indicated that the risk of becoming psychotic was approximately doubled if cannabis dependence was present at intake (Phillips et al. 2001).

Summary of Findings

To date, the best predictors of transition to psychosis remain essentially clinical in nature despite our attempt to enhance the capacity to predict by adding in variables from other domains, such as neurocognitive deficits and developmental milestones. Our clinical experience shows that we have been able to identify and offer assistance to many young people who later demonstrate that they have been in the prodromal phase preceding a first episode of psychosis, as well as to many other young people who turn out to be either true false-positives or false-false-positives. Furthermore, these young people are willing to accept such support and, in most cases, benefit from it. However, they are clearly a help-seeking and help-accepting subgroup of the cohort of young people at risk of serious mental disorders. Moreover, the high rate of transition to psychosis in our study is a cause for concern, even though the existence of the clinic inevitably reduced the duration of untreated psychosis that would otherwise have occurred. The 12-month risk of 40.8% may, in fact, have been higher if the subjects had not attended the PACE Clinic, where they received some treatment. We conclude that more specific treatment needs to be developed to more effectively reduce the risk of transition to psychosis. The nature of such specific treatment clearly remains a research question. It must be acknowledged that numbers to date are small and the findings cannot be generalized to the whole population of people in the prodromal phase of a first psychotic episode.

Some significant predictors of psychosis were found; these are summarized in Table 1–3.

Conclusion

The identification of individuals in the prodromal phase of a first psychotic episode has long been a goal of clinicians and researchers. The possibility of treating these young people before the serious disruption of florid psychosis is the major motivation behind this search. An indicated prevention strategy is likely to have major benefits for the person, his or

Table 1–3.   Predictors of psychosis in PACE Clinic sample

Duration of symptoms greater than 900 days

Global Assessment of Functioning score less than 51

Brief Psychiatric Rating Scale total score greater than 15

Brief Psychiatric Rating Scale psychotic subscale score greater than 2

Scale for the Assessment of Negative Symptoms attention score greater than 1

Hamilton Rating Scale for Depression score greater than 18

Normal left hippocampal volume

Cannabis dependence

Maternal age more than 30 years

her family, and other social networks and to be cost effective as well as humane. Such a paradigm shift represents a major challenge and opens up a whole range of questions. It is wise to proceed slowly on the path to reform. It is vital that reform in clinical practice be based on solid evidence, and this can only be obtained through careful and adequately funded research. If this does not occur, then the enthusiasm will rapidly dissipate, and achievable prevention will become discredited again. On the other hand, we must not let irrational fears inhibit us in collecting the evidence, because the stakes are high. Preventive intervention in psychosis is fundamentally the same as in other physical and mental disorders. The young people at risk are not from another planet. In our experience, they are quite capable of participating in clinical care and clinical research in an informed way. Importantly, we have not witnessed any harm to them deriving from such participation; rather, they have generally benefited substantially. The PACE approach is only one strategy attempting to tackle the problem. To date, we have established that it is possible to identify impending psychosis prospectively, and we have found some factors that predict an increased likelihood of the development of psychosis within our UHR group. The next step is to investigate whether particular interventions can reduce the transition rate among the high-risk group and determine which treatments are most effective. A randomized controlled trial of low-dose neuroleptic agents and cognitive–behavioral therapy in the PACE group is currently underway. It is hoped that this will shed more light on these issues and pave the way for the benefits that indicated prevention has to offer.

References

Allen JJ, Chapman LJ, Chapman JP, et al: Prediction of psychoticlike symptoms in hypothetically psychosis-prone college students. J Abnorm Psychol 96:83–88, 1987

American Psychiatric Association: Diagnostic and Statistical Manual of Mental Disorders, 3rd Edition Revised. Washington, DC, American Psychiatric Association, 1987

American Psychiatric Association: Diagnostic and Statistical Manual of Mental Disorders, 4th Edition. Washington, DC, American Psychiatric Association, 1994

Andreasen N: Negative symptoms in schizophrenia: definition and reliability. Arch Gen Psychiatry 39:784–788, 1982

Andreasen NC, Flaum M, Arndt S: The Comprehensive Assessment of Symptoms and History (CASH): an instrument for assessing diagnosis and psychopathology. Arch Gen Psychiatry 49:615–623, 1992

Army Individual Test Battery, in Manual of Directions and Scoring. Washington, DC, War Department Adjutant General's Office, 1944

Asarnow JR: Children at risk for schizophrenia: converging lines of evidence. Schizophr Bull 14:613–631, 1988

Bell RQ: Multiple-risk cohorts and segmenting risk as solutions to the problem of false positives in risk for the major psychoses. Psychiatry 55:370–381, 1992

Beiser M, Erikson D, Fleming JAE, et al: Establishing the onset of psychotic illness. Am J Psychiatry 150:1349–1354, 1993

Benton AL, Hamsher K: Multilingual Aphasia Examination. Iowa City, IA, AJA Associates, 1983

Birchwood M: Early intervention in schizophrenia: theoretical background and clinical strategies. Br J Clin Psychol 31:257–278, 1992

Birchwood M, Smith J, Macmillan F, et al: Predicting relapse in schizophrenia: the development and implementation of an early signs monitoring system using patients and families as observers: a preliminary investigation. Psychol Med 19:649–656, 1989

Cameron DE: Early schizophrenia. Am J Psychiatry 95:567–578, 1938

Cannon-Spoor HE, Potkin SG, Wyatt RJ: Measurement of premorbid adjustment in chronic schizophrenia. Schizophr Bull 8:470–484, 1982

Chapman LJ, Chapman JP: Scales for rating psychotic and psychoticlike experiences as continua. Schizophr Bull 6:476–489, 1980

Chapman LJ, Chapman JP: The search for symptoms predictive of schizophrenia. Schizophr Bull 13:497–503, 1987

Chapman LJ, Chapman JP, Kwapil TR, et al: Putatively psychosis-prone subjects 10 years later. J Abnorm Psychol 103:171–183, 1994

Claridge G: "The schizophrenias as nervous types" revisited. Br J Psychiatry 151:735–743, 1987

Eaton WW, Badawi M, Melton B: Prodromes and precursors: epidemiologic data for primary prevention of disorders with slow onset. Am J Psychiatry 152:967–972, 1995

Erlenmeyer-Kimling L, Squires-Wheeler E, Adamo UH, et al: The New York High Risk Project: psychoses and cluster A personality disorders in offspring of schizophrenic parents at 23 years of follow-up. Arch Gen Psychiatry 52:857–865, 1995

First MB, Spitzer RL, Gibbon M, et al: Structured Clinical Interview for DSM-IV Axis I Disorders, patient edition (SCID-I/P, Version 2.0). New York, Biometrics Research Department, 1996

Gordon RS: An operational classification of disease prevention. Public Health Rep 98:107–109, 1983

Gottesman II, Shields J: Schizophrenia: the epigenetic puzzle. Cambridge, Cambridge University Press, 1982

Häfner H, Riecher-Rössler A, Hambrect M, et al: IRAOS: an instrument for the assessment of onset and early course of schizophrenia. Schizophr Bull 6:209–223, 1992

Häfner H, Maurer K, Löffler W, et al: The influence of age and sex on the onset and early course of schizophrenia. Br J Psychiatry 162:80–86, 1993

Häfner H, Maurer W, Löffler, B, et al: Onset and early course of schizophrenia, in Causes of Schizophrenia. Edited by Häfner H, Gattaz WF. New York, Springer, 1995a

Häfner H, Nowotny B, Löffler W, et al: When and how does schizophrenia produce social deficits? Eur Arch Psychiatry Clin Neurosci 246:17–28, 1995b

Häfner H, Maurer K, Löffler W, et al: The ABC Schizophrenia Study: a preliminary overview of the results. Soc Psychiatry Psychiatr Epidemiol 33:380–386, 1998

Hamilton M: The assessment of anxiety states by rating. Br J Psychiatry 32:50–55, 1959

Hamilton M: A rating scale for depression. J Neurol Neurosurg Psychiatry 23:56–62, 1960

Heaton RK, Chelune GJ, Talley JL, et al: The Wisconsin Card Sorting Test Manual, revised and expanded. Odessa, Psychological Assessment Resources, 1993

Heinrichs DW, Carpenter WT: Prospective study of prodromal symptoms in schizophrenic relapse. Am J Psychiatry 142:371–373, 1985

Heinrichs D, Hanlon T, Carpenter W: The Quality of Life Scale: an instrument for rating the schizophrenia deficit syndrome. Schizophr Bull 10:388–398, 1984

Herz MI, Melville C: Relapse in schizophrenia. Am J Psychiatry 137:801–805, 1980

Hodges A, Byrne M, Grant E, et al: People at risk of schizophrenia: sample characteristic of the first 100 cases in the Edinburgh High-Risk Study. Br J Psychiatry 174:547–553, 1999

Huber G, Gross G, Shuttler R, et al: Longitudinal studies of schizophrenic patients. Schizophr Bull 6:592–605, 1980

Jackson HJ, McGorry PD, Dudgeon P: Prodromal symptoms of schizophrenia in first episode psychosis: prevalence and specificity. Comp Psychiatry 36:241–250, 1995

Johnstone EC, Abukmeil SS, Byrne M, et al: Edinburgh high risk study—findings after four years: demographic, attainment, and psychopathological issues. Schizophr Res 46:1–15, 2000

Jones P, Bebbington P, Foerster A, et al: Premorbid social underachievement in schizophrenia: results from the Camberwell Collaborative Psychosis Study. Br J Psychiatry 162:65–71, 1993

Jones P, Rodgers B, Murray R, Marmot M: Child development risk factors for adult schizophrenia in the British 1946 birth cohort. Lancet 344:1398–1402, 1994

Keith SJ, Matthews SM: The diagnosis of schizophrenia: a review of onset and duration issues. Schizophr Bull 17:51–67, 1991

Kety SS, Rosenthal D, Wender PH, et al: Mental illness in the biological and adoptive families of adoptive individuals who have become schizophrenic: a preliminary report based on psychiatric interviews, in Genetic Research in Psychiatry. Edited by Rieve RR, Rosenthal D, Brill H. Baltimore, MD, John Hopkins University Press, 1975

Klosterkötter J, Ebel H, Schultze-Lutter F, et al: Diagnostic validity of basic symptoms. Eur Arch Psychiatry Clin Neurosci 246:147–154, 1996

Klosterkötter J, Schultze-Lutter F, Gross G, et al: Early self-experienced neuropsychological deficits and subsequent schizophrenic diseases: an 8-year average follow-up prospective study. Acta Psychiatr Scand 95:396–404, 1997

Klosterkötter J, Hellmich M, Steinmeyer EM, et al: Diagnosing schizophrenia in the initial prodromal phase. Arch Gen Psychiatry 58:158–164, 2001

Krausz M, Muller-Thomsen TSO: Schizophrenia with onset in adolescence: an 11-year followup. Schizophr Bull 19:831–841, 1993

Larsen TK, McGlashan TH, Moe LC: First-episode schizophrenia, I: early course parameters. Schizophr Bull 22:241–256, 1996

Lawrie SM, Whalley H, Kestelman JN, et al: Magnetic resonance imaging of brain in people at high risk of developing schizophrenia. Lancet 353:30–33, 1999

Lewis SW, Owen MJ, Murray RM: Obstetric complications and schizophrenia: methodology and mechanisms, in Schizophrenia: Scientific Progress. Edited by Schultz SC, Tamminga CA. New York, Oxford University Press, 1989

Lezak MD: Neuropsychological Assessment. New York, Oxford University Press, 1995

Loebel AD, Lieberman JA, Alvir JM, et al: Duration of psychosis and outcome in first-episode schizophrenia. Am J Psychiatry 149:1183–1188, 1992

Loranger AW: Personality Disorders Examination (PDE) Manual. Yonkers, NY, DV Communications, 1988

Lukoff D, Liberman RP, Nuechterlein KH: Symptom monitoring in the rehabilitation of schizophrenic patients. Schizophr Bull 12:578–602, 1986

Maxwell ME: Manual for the FIGS. Clinical Neurogenetics Branch, Intramural Research Branch, National Institute of Mental Health, USA, unpublished

McGorry PD, Singh BS: Schizophrenia: risk and possibility, in Handbook of Preventive Psychiatry. Edited by Raphael B, Burrows GD. Amsterdam, Elsevier, 1995

McGorry PD, McFarlane C, Patton GC, et al: The prevalence of prodromal features of schizophrenia in adolescence: a preliminary survey. Acta Psychiatr Scand 90:375–378, 1995

Meares A: The diagnosis of prepsychotic schizophrenia. Lancet i:55–59, 1959

Mednick SA, Parnas J, Schulsinger F: The Copenhagen High-Risk Project, 1962–1986. Schizophr Bull 13:485–496, 1987

Meehl PE: Schizotaxia revisited. Arch Gen Psychiatry 46:935–944, 1989

Mihalopolous C, McGorry PD, Carter RC: Is early intervention in first episode psychosis an economically viable method of improving outcome? Acta Psychiatr Scand 54:1–9, 1999

Mrazek PJ, Haggerty RJ: Reducing Risks for Mental Disorders: Frontiers for Preventive Intervention Research. Washington DC, National Academy Press, 1994

Nelson HE, Willison JR: The Revised National Adult Reading Test—Test Manual. Windsor, United Kingdom, NFER, 1991

Overall JE, Gorham DR: The Brief Psychiatric Rating Scale. Psychol Rep 10:799–812, 1962

Phillips LJ, McGorry PD, Yung AR, et al: Cannabis use and prediction of psychosis. Schizophr Res 49:20, 2001

Phillips LJ, Velahoulis D, Pantelis L, et al: Nonreduction in hippocampal volume is associated with higher risk of psychosis. Under review

Subotnik KL, Nuechterlein KH: Prodromal signs and symptoms of schizophrenic relapse. J Abnorm Psychol 97:405–412, 1988

Sullivan HS: The onset of schizophrenia. Am J Psychiatry 6:105–134, 1927

Tarrier N, Barrowclough C, Bamrah JS: Prodromal signs of relapse in schizophrenia. Soc Psychiatry Psychiatr Epidemiol 26:157–161, 1991

van Os J, Hanssen M, Ravelli A: Strauss (1969) revisited: a psychosis continuum in the general population? Schizophr Res 45:11–20, 2000

Verdoux H, van Os J, Maurice-Tison S, et al: Is early adulthood a critical developmental stage for psychosis proneness? a survey of delusional ideation in normal subjects. Schizophr Res 29:247–254, 1998

Wechsler D: Wechsler Memory Scale, Revised. New York, Psychological Corporation, 1987

Wing JK, Babor T, Brugha T, et al: SCAN: Schedules for clinical assessment in neuropsychiatry. Arch Gen Psychiatry 47:589–593, 1990

Young RC, Biggs JT, Ziegler VE, et al: A rating scale for mania: reliability, validity and sensitivity. Br J Psychiatry 133:429–435, 1978

Yung AR, Jackson HJ: The onset of psychotic disorder: clinical and research aspects, in The Recognition and Management of Early Psychosis: A Preventive Approach. Edited by McGorry PD, Jackson HJ. New York, Cambridge University Press, 1999

Yung AR, McGorry PD: The initial prodrome in psychosis: descriptive and qualitative aspects. Aust NZ J Psychiatry 30:587–599, 1996

Yung AR, McGorry PD, McFarlane CA, et al: Monitoring and care of young people at incipient risk of psychosis. Schizophr Bull 22:283–303, 1996

Yung AR, Phillips LJ, McGorry PD, et al: Can we predict first episode psychosis in a high risk group? Int Clin Psychopharm 13(suppl 1):23–30, 1998a

Yung AR, Phillips LJ, McGorry PD, et al: The prediction of psychosis: a step towards indicated prevention of schizophrenia? Br J Psychiatry 172(suppl 33):14–20, 1998b

Yung AR, Yuen HP, Phillips LJ, et al: Psychosis prediction: 12 month follow-up of a high risk ('prodromal') group. Schizophr Res, under review

Epidemiology of First-Episode Schizophrenia

The Suffolk County Mental Health Project

Evelyn J. Bromet, Ph.D.

Ramin Mojtabai, M.D., Ph.D.

Shmuel Fennig, M.D.

Since the early 1900s, hundreds—if not thousands—of follow-up studies have presented findings on the course and outcome of schizophrenia and other major psychiatric and substance use disorders. These studies have two fundamental purposes. The first is to describe the morbidity patterns associated with specific diagnoses, and the second is to identify the biopsychosocial predictors of better and worse outcome. Wide variability has been observed in the patterns of morbidity, defined as rehospitaliza-

We gratefully acknowledge the contribution of many collaborators to the study, particularly Drs. Gabrielle Carlson, Thomas J. Craig, Marsha Karant, and Joseph E. Schwartz. Janet Lavelle, project coordinator, has been invaluable in overseeing all aspects of the project. We are especially grateful to the participants and their families for sharing their time and insights with us. This research has been supported by National Institute of Mental Health Grant MH44801.

tion, clinical relapse, symptom exacerbation, or deterioration in psychosocial functioning, and few prognostic variables have been consistently identified from one study to the other.

Because there are major differences in how the studies were designed, it is not surprising that the findings have been inconsistent. Some of the important methodological decisions that can affect the ultimate findings are listed in Table 2–1. One fundamental issue is the nature of the sample itself. Is the sample based on consecutive-admission or first-admission patients? Consecutive admissions include a mixture of chronically ill treatment seekers as well as individuals with recent onsets. The group outcome rates vary substantially depending on the proportion of chronically ill to recently ill individuals in a given sample (Cohen and Cohen 1984). First-admission samples are also heterogeneous with respect to whether the patient is experiencing a true first episode or has had prior treated or untreated episodes.

Another basic issue is whether the sample was drawn from a single site or from multiple facilities and whether the facilities are representative of where most patients are treated or are special tertiary-care facilities. Many follow-up studies are conducted in a single academic or veterans' hospital facility. Patients are often referred to such centers because they have complex histories and are difficult to diagnose and treat. It has also been documented that clinical research units located in academic facilities tend to admit relatively few minority patients (Adebimpe 1994); hence, there is a racial and corresponding socioeconomic bias in study subjects selected from these settings. Ironically, the prevalence data clearly show an inverse relationship between socioeconomic status and schizophrenia (Dohrenwend et al. 1992; Eaton et al. 1988); therefore, many follow-up samples are not representative of patients with a given disease. A few studies, such as the Collaborative Depression Project (e.g., Coryell 1990a and 1990b), sampled patients from more than one facility; but even these studies were typically restricted to academic centers. Aside from the Vancouver (Beiser et al. 1993) and World Health Organization's (Leff et al. 1992) programs of research on schizophrenia and recent studies using case registry samples, there are few examples of studies that draw patients from a representative sample of treatment settings, particularly in the United States.

Other sampling decisions also affect the comparability of findings. Some samples consist of volunteers rather than subjects who were systematically selected. Some samples exclude patients with serious substance abuse histories, usually because such patients present diagnostic

Table 2–1. Methodological variations in follow-up studies

Sample

First versus consecutive admission

First admission versus first-episode cases

If first admission, prior medication treatment as exclusion variable

Volunteer versus systematic sampling

High versus low response rate

Comorbid substance abuse versus no comorbidity

Age distribution criteria

All admissions or only those living with family member

Single hospital versus multiple settings

Representative settings versus academic or Veterans' Affairs hospital only

Diagnosis

Chart review versus structured interview

Cross-sectional versus longitudinal

Consensus diagnosis or individual psychiatrist's diagnosis

Structured interview used

DSM versus ICD

Treatment experiences

Protocol driven or naturalistic

Nature of follow-up treatment

Type of medications (may vary by region)

Follow-up issues

Clinical background (if any) of the interviewer

Timing of follow-up

Length of follow-up

Number of follow-up contacts

Telephone versus face-to-face interview

Domains measured

Selection of scales

Definitions of poor outcome

Attrition in the sample

and management problems. Because of the pervasiveness of substance use problems in patients treated in mental health clinics, findings from studies with this exclusion criterion are not generalizable to the universe of individuals with serious mental disorders.

Convincing people with schizophrenia to participate in research presents a great challenge, and a low initial response rate and a high attrition rate over the follow-up period also contribute to sampling bias. Many studies are biased toward including cooperative patients rather than those who are difficult to diagnose (often because of substance abuse).

Another factor that makes it difficult to compare the course of illness across studies is diagnosis. The issue is not simply the classification system used to formulate the diagnosis, but how the information was gathered to make that judgment in the first place. Was the information gathered systematically, through a structured interview combined with all other sources of information, or was it based only on a review of medical records or other available clinical evidence? Was it based only on cross-sectional and retrospective data, or was longitudinal information incorporated? Was it formulated on the basis of a single structured interview without integrating other sources of information?

In the past, when chart reviews and clinical diagnoses were the mainstay of follow-up research, the clinical diagnosis was often deferred while the patient was observed over the course of several weeks of hospitalization. Thus, in effect, the clinical diagnosis was a longitudinal decision. With the shortened duration of hospital stays, clinicians no longer have this luxury, and research that uses the diagnosis in the medical record or discharge summary reflects this reduced degree of precision. This is an especially important issue in studies of first-admission patients. In such studies, even if the diagnosis is based on an amalgam of structured interview and medical record information, the sample may include false-positives (i.e., people who initially fit the diagnostic criteria but later are found to have been misclassified) and false-negatives (i.e., people who do not meet the criteria initially but later do). The study described here chose to mimic the clinical process and formulate a research diagnosis longitudinally, using all available information gathered over the 2-year period after the first hospitalization.

Another factor that affects the comparability of the results is whether the study population was part of a clinical treatment protocol. It is clear that consistent drug treatment is the best predictor of outcome in schizophrenia (Wyatt et al. 1998). Patients who agree to participate in a drug study often do better while they are taking the medication and taking part in the intensive activities associated with being a study participant. Thus, Loebel et al. (1992) showed very good initial outcomes in patients who were part of a treatment protocol, but a few years after the treatment protocol ended, the relapse rate was extremely high (Robinson et al. 1999). Patients participating in drug trials are also different in other respects:

they are more cooperative, able to handle a washout period, and can often be stabilized before random assignment.

Table 2–1 also lists other methodological decisions about follow-up strategies that vary across studies and reduce our ability to make cross-study comparisons. These include timing and length of the follow-up period, the qualifications of the follow-up raters, the choice of measures, how the longitudinal data were obtained (e.g., face-to-face interviews, telephone contact, registry information), and attrition in the sample. Variations in course and outcome measures also diminish our ability to compare results across these studies.

Epidemiology provides a framework that minimizes the bias in follow-up research. One of the fundamental features of an epidemiologic study is assembling a representative cohort of patients (Ram et al. 1992). Attention is given to selecting representative treatment facilities as well as unbiased samples of patients within facilities. The most informative clinical sample identifies patients at the onset of their illness. In psychiatry, although first-episode patients are optimal for understanding remission and relapse over time, first-admission patients provide the most practical means of assembling a newly diagnosed cohort. Of course, the ideal strategy is to identify groups before or during the prodromal stage, but this is difficult to achieve except in studies of high-risk samples. However, high-risk samples are not necessarily representative of patients with a given disorder.

In 1989, we began an epidemiologic study of the course of illness in patients with psychotic symptoms selected at the time of their first hospitalization (Bromet et al. 1992). This ongoing study identified subjects from each of the inpatient treatment facilities in Suffolk County (Long Island, New York) and therefore provides data on one of the most representative samples ever assembled. We focused special attention on the stability of the diagnosis; the comparison of illness course by diagnosis; and the predictors of illness course including age, gender, substance abuse, suicide history, premorbid social competence, illness duration and severity, and treatment. When our study was conceived, no systematic information was available regarding the distribution of diagnoses in such a sample, the stability of the initial clinical or research diagnosis, or how patients with different diagnoses would fare over time. Indeed, there were very few first-admission studies of patients with affective psychosis, and none used a systematic, longitudinal approach to diagnosis.

Design of the Suffolk County
Mental Health Project

The Suffolk County study assembled a cohort of 674 first-admission patients recruited from the 12 inpatient facilities in Suffolk County, Long Island, New York (population, 1.3 million), from 1989 to 1995 who were believed to have psychotic symptoms. The settings included an adult and a child state hospital, a veterans' hospital with multiple psychiatric wards, a 30-bed academic inpatient ward, six 20–30-bed community hospital wards, and two psychiatric facilities (added in 1994). In each site, the head nurse or social worker or a project staff member identified potential study participants using the following inclusion criteria: age 15–60 years, resident of Suffolk County, and clinical evidence of psychosis or a facility diagnosis indicating psychosis. Patients were excluded if they were unwilling to give informed consent, their first lifetime psychiatric hospitalization occurred more than 6 months before the index admission, the psychosis had a clear organic etiology (except substance abuse), or they were deemed noninterviewable because of significant mental retardation or inability to speak English. Thus, although the sample is more representative than other first-admission samples in the United States to date, it should be noted that patients who did not seek inpatient care, were treated outside of Suffolk County, were treated only in the emergency room or jail, or could not participate in an interview were not included in the sample.

Patients were approached for the study after their psychosis had cleared in order to meet human subject guidelines for capacity to consent. Thus, most interviews took place in the hospital shortly before discharge and well after treatment was initiated. The initial response rate was 72%; more than 85% of the respondents were successfully followed up with over a 2-year period. Many retention strategies were implemented to maintain as high a follow-up rate as possible, including maintaining consistent interviewers, having contact with respondents every 3 months, updating location information at each major contact with respondents or significant others, offering a financial incentive, scheduling interviews at times and places convenient to the respondents, and dropping by the respondents' homes if necessary to schedule interviews. Additionally, we routinely mailed the patients birthday cards and holiday cards.

The interviewers were experienced master's-level mental health professionals who were consistent with the requirements of administering a semistructured diagnostic instrument. Follow-up interviews were not done blindly because the major goal of the study was to obtain accurate information and reconcile discrepancies rather than provide further confirmation of the inconsistency of people's reports over time. In fact, the interviewers were explicitly instructed to review previous clinical information so they could disentangle discrepancies if they occurred during the follow-up interviews. The respondent's research diagnosis was the only variable concealed from the interviewer.

Assessment Tools

The baseline assessment focused primarily on diagnosis using the Structured Clinical Interview for DSM-III-R (SCID; Spitzer et al. 1992). Subsequently, respondents were recontacted every 3 months by telephone, and face-to-face interviews were done at 6, 24, and 48 months' follow-up. At each face-to-face follow-up interview, an interval SCID, the Quality of Life Scale (Heinrichs et al. 1984), and questionnaires on treatment experiences and treatment satisfaction were administered. At the 6-month follow-up, detailed information on premorbid functioning was obtained in order to complete the Premorbid Adjustment Scale (Cannon-Spoor et al. 1982). In addition, after each face-to-face assessment, the interviewers completed the Brief Psychiatric Rating Scale (BPRS; Woerner et al. 1988), the Scale for the Assessment of Negative Symptoms (SANS; Andreasen 1983), the Scale for the Assessment of Positive Symptoms (SAPS; Andreasen 1984), the Hamilton Rating Scale for Depression (HRSD; Hamilton 1960), and the Global Assessment of Functioning (GAF). Discharge summaries were requested for all hospitalizations.

Research Diagnosis

The research diagnoses were based on a review of pertinent diagnostic information, including medical record discharge summaries, clinical information from the medical record recorded by the interviewer, significant other interviews, the SCID, school records, and structured narratives written by the interviewers after each contact. The SCID was modified by omitting the skip-out rules for the depression and mania modules and adding items on violence, suicidal behavior, and quantity and frequency of substance use. Symptoms documented only in the medical record were given a special code. The interviewers' narratives summarized the respondent's psychiatric, occupational, and psychosocial functioning, including major life events and treatment.

A longitudinal research diagnosis was formulated after the 6- and 24-month follow-up interviews. Pairs of psychiatrists independently reviewed all of the clinical material delineated, assigned a diagnosis, and completed DSM criteria checklists developed for the project to enhance reliability (Fennig et al. 1994). Each case was then discussed by the two psychiatrists. Regardless of whether they agreed on the diagnosis, all cases were presented at monthly meetings of four or more psychiatrists. At these meetings, primary and comorbid consensus diagnoses were assigned using both DSM-III-R (American Psychiatric Association 1987) and DSM-IV (American Psychiatric Association 1994) criteria. At these meetings, we reached a consensus about whether the diagnosis was definite or probable (i.e., the person did not quite reach criteria but everyone agreed that this was the most likely diagnosis). The previous research diagnosis was revealed to the group after the consensus decision was reached. If the new diagnosis was different from the previous one, the psychiatrists then determined what factors accounted for the change (i.e., illness course, new information not previously known, reinterpretation of the same information).

Results and Comments

Characteristics of the Sample

The patients were sampled from the adult state hospital (31%), university ward (33%), and community or private facilities (33%), with a handful of patients (3%) hospitalized at the veterans' hospital or the child state facility. Table 2–2 presents the demographic characteristics of the sample. The sample was predominantly male (59%), white (75%), and unmarried (64%). According to the 1990 census, slightly more than 90% of the Suffolk County population was white. One quarter of the sample had been in a special education program. With respect to age, 23% were 15–21 at the time of their admission, 32% were 22–29, and 45% were 30 years and older. The median duration of psychosis before hospitalization was 39 days. The range was from patients who were hospitalized on the day their psychosis began to patients who experienced their first psychotic symptom more than 22 years before the admission. One-third of the patients was hospitalized within 14 days, one-third was hospitalized from 14 days to 6 months, and one-third (primarily with schizophrenia) was hospitalized more than 6 months after the first psychotic symptom. (For a more detailed analysis of duration of untreated psychosis in the sample, see Craig et al. 2000.)

Table 2–2. Characteristics of the Suffolk County sample (*N*=674)

Characteristics	Median
Age (years)	28
Days from onset of psychosis to first hospitalization	39
Gender	
Male	58.6%
Female	41.4%
Race	
White	75.1%
Black	15.3%
Hispanic	6.7%
Other	3.0%
Marital status	
Never married	63.9%
Current married or living as if married	20.1%
Divorced or separated	14.9%
Widowed	0.9%
Education	
Less than high school	22.9%
High school graduate	34.9%
More than high school	42.2%
Special education placement	25.4%
Household occupation	
White collar	53.2%
Blue collar	46.8%

Slightly more than half (52%) of the sample had a history of lifetime alcohol or drug abuse or dependence. The lifetime suicide attempt rate was 28%. Consistent with findings from general population samples, there was a significant relationship between substance abuse and suicide attempts, with 34% of respondents with a history of substance abuse or dependence having made a suicide attempt compared with 22.6% of those without a history of substance abuse (χ^2=10.2; P<0.001).

Most of the study subjects (89%; n=600) were initially interviewed at the time of their first lifetime hospitalization. A total of 11% (n=74) had their first lifetime hospitalization in the previous 6 months, usually outside of Suffolk County. There were no demographic or diagnostic (including substance abuse) differences or differences in subsequent treatment experiences between the 600 patients selected at the time of their first hospitalization and the 74 with a hospitalization in the previous 6 months. However, as expected, the previously hospitalized patients were more likely to report prior psychotropic drug use. Specifically, 63% of the previously hospitalized versus 14% of the first-hospitalized patients received antipsychotic medications before the baseline hospitalization, and 43% versus 22% received other psychiatric medications ($P<0.001$ for both variables).

Diagnostic Distribution

At the 6-month follow-up interview, when the first longitudinal research diagnosis was formulated, sufficient longitudinal information was available for 603 subjects. The largest diagnostic category was schizophrenia (24%), followed by bipolar disorder with psychotic features (23%) and major depressive disorder with psychotic features (14%; Table 2–3).

Table 2–3. Distribution of consensus research diagnoses at 6- and 24-month follow-up

DSM-IV diagnosis	At 6 months, %	At 24 months, %	Same diagnosis at 24 months, %
Schizophrenia	24.2	31.4	91.4
Schizoaffective disorder	5.8	5.0	35.3
Schizophreniform disorder	2.0	1.2	54.5
Bipolar disorder with psychotic features	22.9	23.1	80.7
Major depressive disorder with psychotic features	13.8	14.3	73.8
Brief psychotic episode	1.8	1.5	27.3
Psychosis not otherwise specified	4.8	4.2	40.0
Delusional disorder	1.3	1.8	57.1
Substance diagnosis	6.8	6.8	65.7
Unknown	4.0	2.7	9.1
Organic (not substance related)	2.0	1.5	80.0
Questionable or not psychotic	10.6	6.3	55.3

Note. Because of missing longitudinal information, 6-month consensus diagnoses were formulated for 603 members of the cohort and 24-month diagnoses were made for 601 patients. A total of 551 were diagnosed at both times.

At 24-month follow-up, diagnoses were assigned for 601 subjects with sufficiently detailed longitudinal information. Again, the largest diagnostic category was schizophrenia (31%), followed by bipolar disorder with psychotic features (23%) and major depressive disorder with psychotic features (14%). Thus, there was a marked shift into the category of schizophrenia between 6- and 24-month follow-up.

Although many respondents received the same diagnosis at each of these times, there were a number of discrepancies across time in the research diagnosis, caused primarily by illness course and, less frequently, by new disclosures that were previously unknown. The last column of Table 2–3 shows the extent to which people remained in the same category at 24-month follow-up. These percentages were calculated only for the 551 individuals who were diagnosed at both 6- and 24-month follow-up. The most stable category was schizophrenia—that is, among respondents receiving the diagnosis of schizophrenia at 6-month follow-up, 91% received the same diagnosis 18 months later. The next most stable categories were bipolar disorder with psychotic features (81%) and organic psychosis (80%). The least stable, not surprisingly, were psychosis not otherwise specified (40%) and unknown diagnosis at 6 months (9%).

As noted previously, the biggest shift we observed was into the schizophrenia spectrum category. Schwartz et al. (2000) conducted a series of analyses to identify the predictors of shifting from a diagnosis outside the schizophrenia spectrum at 6-month follow-up to a 24-month schizophrenia diagnosis in the Suffolk County cohort. The risk factors included being given a clinical diagnosis of schizophrenia by the admitting facility, being discharged from the admitting facility while taking antipsychotic medication, having a longer initial duration of stay, having poorer psychosocial adjustment during adolescence, having a life history of substance disorder, and having high negative symptoms at 6-month follow-up. Although the change in diagnosis was mostly attributable to the evolution of the illness, our rigid adherence to the DSM-IV requirements may have also played a role in our failure to diagnose people with schizophrenia with the available evidence at hand.

Prehospital Differences Between Schizophrenia and Nonorganic Psychoses

Before the baseline assessment, respondents with 24-month diagnoses of schizophrenia, schizoaffective disorder, and schizophreniform disorder ($n=226$) differed ($P<0.001$) on a number of variables from those diagnosed with other nonorganic psychoses (e.g., affective psychosis, psychosis not otherwise specified, delusional disorder, brief psychotic episode; $n=271$). Specifically, the group with schizophrenia was significantly more likely to have been in special education classes (35% vs. 21% of the other psychosis group), to be younger (median age = 26 vs. 29 years), to be male (65% vs. 47%), and to have experienced their first psychotic symptom earlier (median = 223 days vs. 15 days before first hospitalization).

Compared with the other psychosis group, the premorbid adjustment of the schizophrenia group was significantly poorer at each of the three age periods covered by the Cannon-Spoor rating scale (i.e., 6–11, 12–15, and 16–18). Moreover, the schizophrenia group's functioning declined with age (mean±SD for schizophrenia: 0.32±0.17, 0.35±0.18, 0.40±0.19; higher scores indicate worse functioning). By comparison, those of the other psychosis group were more stable (0.26±0.16, 0.28±0.16, and 0.29±0.16). A repeated measures analysis of variance revealed significant main effects for diagnosis and age and a significant diagnosis by age interaction ($P<0.001$).

Similarly, the baseline GAF rating for the best month of the year before hospitalization was significantly poorer for individuals with schizophrenia (mean±SD = 52.3±13.7) than for those with other psychoses (64.0±12.7). Because the psychosis itself began before this 1-year period in many individuals with schizophrenia, the analysis was repeated, controlling for duration of psychosis before hospitalization using analysis of covariance. The difference remained highly significant ($P<0.001$).

Thus, respondents diagnosed with schizophrenia were at a psychosocial disadvantage before they ever reached the hospital. We now examine how this affected their later functioning.

Diagnostic Differences in Posthospital Functioning

In a previous paper (Bromet et al. 1996), we presented differences by diagnosis in the 6-month outcomes of the first half of the cohort, showing that those with schizophrenia functioned more poorly in the first 6-month follow-up period than both the bipolar and depressed psychosis groups. Here we extend the findings to the 24-month follow-up period and include the entire sample.

Table 2–4 shows that the pattern of results at 24-month follow-up was similar to that previously reported for the 6-month period. Thus, individuals with schizophrenia had significantly poorer psychosocial functioning as measured by the GAF, Quality of Life scales (0 [poor] to 6 [good]), positive and negative symptoms, thought disturbance, and depression severity (although both groups were at the low end of the HRSD). They were also more likely to exhibit psychotic symptoms during the 24-month interview, to have received treatment in the past 6 months (before the 24-month interview), and to have been rehospitalized between baseline and 24-month follow-up.

Table 2–4. Diagnostic differences in functioning at 24-month follow-up

24-month variable*	Schizophrenia, mean (SD)	Other psychosis, mean (SD)
Global Assessment of Functioning: best month between 6 and 24 months	49.1 (12.7)	66.0 (12.7)
Hamilton Rating Scale for Depression	8.2 (5.5)	5.7 (5.5)
Brief Psychiatric Rating Scale: thought disturbance	1.7 (0.7)	1.3 (0.7)
Scale for the Assessment of Negative Symptoms: negative symptom severity	1.8 (.9)	0.7 (0.7)
Scale for the Assessment of Positive Symptoms: positive symptom severity	0.8 (0.8)	0.3 (0.6)
Quality of Life: household intimacy	4.3 (1.7)	5.0 (1.2)
Quality of Life: relations with friends	2.7 (1.2)	3.7 (1.2)
Quality of Life: social activity	2.8 (1.6)	4.3 (1.6)
Quality of Life: role impairment	2.7 (1.2)	4.1 (1.7)
	Patients, %	Patients, %
Psychotic during 24-month interview	38.0	9.6
Received treatment around 24-month point	78.2	60.0
Rehospitalized during follow-up period	49.6	33.6

Note. All variables were significantly different at $P<0.001$. SD = standard deviation.
*Higher scores indicate better functioning on the Global Assessment of Functioning and Quality of Life scales and poorer functioning on all other measures.

Change Between Prehospital and Posthospital Global Assessment of Functioning Scores

Because the GAF score for the best level of functioning was significantly correlated with each of the other outcome variables (correlations ranged from $r=0.43$ with household intimacy to $r=0.73$ with role impairment and -0.73 with the SANS), this variable was selected for examining the extent and direction of change in functioning across time. At baseline, the median GAF scores were 50 and 65 for the schizophrenia and other psychosis groups, respectively. At 24-month follow-up, the median GAF scores were 45 and 70 for these two groups. Thus, whereas the schizophrenia group had an overall decline in functioning over time, the other psychosis group improved. Using paired *t* tests, the changes in functioning were found to be statistically significant ($P=0.003$ for schizophrenia and 0.02 for the other psychosis group).

Diagnostic Differences in Outcome Adjusting for Prehospital Functioning

The two diagnostic groups were compared on the same set of outcome measures using analysis of covariance, controlling for the baseline GAF, the Cannon-Spoor measure of early childhood adjustment, and placement in special education classes. The diagnostic differences remained highly significant for each outcome variable. Thus, even after adjusting for important prehospital differences, the schizophrenia group performed significantly more poorly at follow-up than did individuals with other psychotic disorders.

Diagnosis-Specific Predictors of Change in Global Assessment of Functioning Scores Over Time

We next applied the median GAF value at baseline to create four change groups. In the schizophrenia group, 76 respondents had a GAF ≤50 at both baseline and follow-up (low–low), 53 were above 50 each time (high–high), 20 improved (low–high), and 40 individuals declined (high–low). In the other psychosis group, 74 individuals had a GAF ≤65 at each time (low–low), 78 were above (high–high), 44 improved (low–high), and 30 declined (high–low).

Table 2–5 presents the distribution of the demographic and clinical variables in the other psychosis change groups. Individuals with consistently poor functioning (low–low) were most likely to be from blue collar households and have the poorest childhood adjustment scores on the Cannon-Spoor scale. Individuals with consistently good functioning (high–high) were least likely to come from blue collar homes, to have an insidious onset of their illness, to have more severe negative symptoms at baseline, and to stay in the hospital longer than average (for the type of hospital they were in). Almost everyone in this group had recovered by 6-month follow-up. The two change groups (low–high and high–low) differed only in suicide attempt history (the low–high group was twice as likely to have made a suicide attempt as the high–low group) and in treatment at the 24-month follow-up point (the low-high group were less likely to be receiving treatment).

Table 2–5. Predictors of stability and change in Global Assessment of Functioning scores in patients with other psychoses (affective psychosis, delusional disorder, brief psychosis, psychosis not otherwise specified)

Variable	Low–low (n=74)	Low–high (n=44)	High–low (n=30)	High–high (n=78)	P
Gender (male), %	51.4	36.4	50.0	43.6	NS
Age, *mean (SD)*	30.3 (10.1)	28.2 (8.5)	29.4 (8.9)	30.5 (10.4)	NS
Blue collar household, %	54.3	43.2	46.5	22.7	<0.01
Never married, %	66.2	54.8	48.3	48.6	NS
Special education, %	28.4	20.5	23.3	15.4	NS
Insidious onset (World Health Organization), %	41.7	47.4	52.9	15.8	<0.01
Lifetime substance use disorder, %	56.8	56.8	40.0	37.2	<0.05
Lifetime suicide attempt, %	33.8	34.1	16.7	14.1	0.01
Childhood adjustment, *mean (SD)*	0.32 (.15)	0.27 (.18)	0.27 (.13)	0.19 (.14)	<0.001
Hospital stay greater than median, %	56.9	55.8	55.2	32.9	0.01
Scale for the Assessment of Negative Symptoms baseline score, *mean (SD)*	1.4 (0.8)	1.2 (1.0)	1.0 (0.8)	0.7 (0.7)	<0.001
Scale for the Assessment of Positive Symptoms baseline score, *mean (SD)*	1.6 (0.9)	1.7 (0.8)	1.6 (1.1)	1.6 (0.9)	NS
Brief Psychiatric Rating Scale total, *mean (SD)*	40.3 (9.1)	42.0 (9.6)	39.2 (9.4)	36.5 (9.3)	0.02
Index episode resolved at 6 months, %	64.8	84.1	63.3	92.3	<0.001

Table 2–5. Predictors of stability and change in Global Assessment of Functioning scores in patients with other psychoses (affective psychosis, delusional disorder, brief psychosis, psychosis not otherwise specified) *(continued)*

Variable	Low–low (n=74)	Low–high (n=44)	High–low (n=30)	High–high (n=78)	P
Taking medication at 6-month follow-up, %	72.3	65.1	80.0	67.6	NS
Taking medication at 24-month follow-up, %	65.3	43.9	75.9	56.0	<0.05

Note. Based on a median split on the baseline Global Assessment of Functioning score of 65. Groups were compared using analysis of variance for continuous variables and chi-square for categorical variables. NS=not significant.

Among the patients with schizophrenia (Table 2–6), the stable, high-functioning group (high–high) was least likely to have had an insidious onset of their illness, but no other pre-baseline characteristic was distinguished among the GAF score change groups. At the time of the baseline interview, the stable high-functioning group had the lowest level of negative symptoms and was somewhat less likely to have long hospital stays. By 6-month follow-up, they were more likely to have achieved some form of remission of their index episode compared with those in the other three groups. It should be noted that the 53 high–high respondents included all seven subjects with schizophreniform disorder and 12 of the 26 subjects with schizoaffective disorder.

Conclusions

When we began our study in 1989, there were few first-admission studies of patients with psychosis. There continues to be a striking dearth of follow-up studies of first-admission patients with psychoses other than schizophrenia. This includes a paucity of research on first-admission patients with psychotic affective disorders.

The patterns and predictors of illness course in schizophrenia and other psychoses have rarely been compared directly (Harrow et al. 1997; Vetter and Köller 1996). The available evidence indicates that people with schizophrenia have poorer short- and long-term outcomes than do individuals with other psychosis diagnoses (Bromet et al. 1996; Harrow et al. 1997; Vetter and Köller 1996). This chapter supports this conclusion and further demonstrates that this pattern holds true even after adjusting for important prehospital differences. Moreover, we found that whereas patients with schizophrenia had an overall decline in functioning compared with prehospital levels, those with other psychotic disorders tended to improve.

Coryell et al. (1990a, 1990b) published two parallel studies on psychotic depression and psychotic bipolar disorder and found predictors of poorer outcome that were similar to those identified for schizophrenia—namely, poorer adolescent social functioning and longer duration of index episode. More recently, Strakowski et al. (1998) assessed the 12-month course of first-admission patients with affective psychosis and found that the individuals had great difficulty recovering from their illness and that delayed recovery was significantly predicted by low socioeconomic status, poor premorbid functioning, treatment noncompliance, and substance abuse. Our findings from an epidemiologically-derived

Table 2–6. Predictors of stability and change in Global Assessment of Functioning scores in patients with schizophrenia, schizoaffective disorder, and schizophreniform disorder

Variable	Low–low (n=76)	Low–high (n=20)	High–low (n=40)	High–high (n=53)	P
Gender (male), %	65.8	60.0	70.0	64.2	NS
Age, mean (SD)	29.5 (8.8)	25.8 (6.9)	26.7 (7.7)	27.5 (9.3)	NS
Blue collar household, %	59.4	47.4	52.8	55.3	NS
Never married, %	77.8	89.5	74.4	75.0	NS
Special education, %	41.9	40.0	35.9	32.1	NS
Insidious onset (World Health Organization), %	83.6	80.0	81.6	54.0	<0.02
Lifetime substance use disorder, %	43.4	35.0	52.5	39.6	NS
Lifetime suicide attempt, %	31.6	25.0	27.5	20.8	NS
Childhood adjustment, mean (SD)	0.37 (0.16)	0.32 (0.18)	0.30 (0.18)	0.30 (0.16)	NS
Hospital stay greater than median, %	77.6	70.0	71.1	50.9	0.02
Scale for the Assessment of Negative Symptoms baseline score, mean (SD)	2.2 (0.9)	2.3 (1.0)	1.8 (0.8)	1.6 (0.8)	<0.001
Scale for the Assessment of Positive Symptoms baseline score, mean (SD)	2.1 (0.9)	2.2 (1.1)	1.7 (0.9)	1.9 (1.0)	NS
Brief Psychiatric Rating Scale total, mean (SD)	42.8 (8.9)	41.9 (9.1)	41.2 (9.1)	39.0 (9.5)	NS
Index episode resolved at 6-month follow-up, %	23.7	60.0	30.8	69.8	<0.001

Table 2–6. Predictors of stability and change in Global Assessment of Functioning scores in patients with schizophrenia, schizoaffective disorder, and schizophreniform disorder *(continued)*

Variable	Low–low (*n*=76)	Low–high (*n*=20)	High–low (*n*=40)	High–high (*n*=53)	*P*
Taking medication at 6-month follow-up, %	80.3	75.0	81.6	85.1	NS
Taking medication at 24-month follow-up, %	81.1	89.5	83.8	66.0	<0.10

Note. Based on a median split on the baseline Global Assessment of Functioning score of 50. Groups were compared using analysis of variance for continuous variables and chi-square for categorical variables. NS=not significant.

sample confirmed that premorbid functioning was a predictor of better psychosocial functioning 2 years after the first hospitalization. Future analyses will explore these issues in greater detail, paying special attention to specific nonschizophrenia diagnoses and to the effects of follow-up treatment.

The majority of subjects in our study received treatment during the first 6 months after hospitalization. However, by 2-year follow-up, the percentages had declined considerably. Although some individuals had recovered and no longer needed treatment, some of those not receiving medications or psychotherapy were clearly in need (e.g., 29% of patients with schizophrenia and 4.6% of patients with other psychoses who were not in treatment at 24-month follow-up had current psychotic symptoms). Given the overall decline in functioning of the patients with schizophrenia and the sizeable percentage of other psychosis patients whose functioning did not improve over their pre-baseline level, it seems that more aggressive or at least more prolonged treatment may be of great benefit. Of course, obtaining care is correlated with having some form of health insurance, and obtaining and maintaining health insurance was not always possible for the patients in this sample.

Most clinical studies in psychiatry would benefit from an epidemiologic approach. The ultimate goal is to articulate an unbiased view of illness course and its predictors. This requires sample selection, diagnosis, longitudinal measurement procedures, and empirical testing of models that maximize the study's power to demonstrate effects with the least amount of bias.

References

Adebimpe VR: Race, racism, and epidemiological surveys. Hospital and Community Psychiatry 45:27–31, 1994

American Psychiatric Association: Diagnostic and Statistical Manual of Mental Disorders, 3rd Edition Revised. Washington, DC, American Psychiatric Association, 1987

American Psychiatric Association: Diagnostic and Statistical Manual of Mental Disorders, 4th Edition. Washington, DC, American Psychiatric Association, 1994

Andreasen NC: The Scale for the Assessment of Negative Symptoms (SANS). Iowa City, IA, University of Iowa, 1983

Andreasen NC: The Scale for the Assessment of Positive Symptoms (SAPS). Iowa City, IA, University of Iowa, 1984

Beiser M, Erickson D, Fleming J, et al: Establishing the onset of psychotic illness. Am J Psychiatry 150:1349–1354, 1993

Bromet E, Schwartz J, Fennig S, et al: The epidemiology of psychosis: the Suffolk County Mental Health Project. Schizophr Bull 18:243–255, 1992

Bromet EJ, Jandorf L, Fennig S, et al: The Suffolk County Mental health project: demographic, pre-morbid and clinical correlates of 6 month outcome. Psychol Med 26:953–962, 1996

Cannon-Spoor HE, Potkin SG, Wyatt RG: Measurement of premorbid adjustment in chronic schizophrenia. Schizophr Bull 8:470–484, 1982

Cohen P, Cohen J: The clinician's illusion. Arch Gen Psychiatry 41:1178–1182, 1984

Coryell W, Keller M, Lavori P, et al: Affective syndromes, psychotic features, and prognosis, I: depression. Arch Gen Psychiatry 47:651–657, 1990a

Coryell W, Keller M, Lavori P, et al: Affective syndromes, psychotic features, and prognosis, II: mania. Arch Gen Psychiatry 47:658–662, 1990b

Craig TJ, Bromet EB, Fennig S, et al: Is there an association between duration of untreated psychosis and 24-month clinical outcome in a first-admission series? Am J Psychiatry 157:60–66, 2000

Dohrenwend BP, Levav I, Shrout PE, et al: Socioeconomic status and psychiatric disorders: the causation-selection issue. Science 255:946–952, 1992

Eaton WW, Day R, Kramer M: The use of epidemiology for risk factor research in schizophrenia: an overview and methodologic critique, in Handbook of Schizophrenia, Vol 3: Nosology, Epidemiology and Genetics of Schizophrenia. Edited by Tsuang MT, Simpson JC. New York, Elsevier, 1988, pp 169–204

Fennig S, Kovasznay B, Rich C, et al: Six-month stability of psychiatric diagnosis in first admission patients with psychosis. Am J Psychiatry 151:1200–1208, 1994

Hamilton M: A rating scale for depression. J Neurol Neurosurg Psychiatry 23:56–62, 1960

Harrow M, Sands JR, Silverstein ML, et al: Course and outcome for schizophrenia versus other psychotic patients: a longitudinal study. Schizophr Bull 23:287–303, 1997

Heinrichs DW, Hanlon TE, Carpenter WT Jr: The Quality of Life Scale: an instrument for rating the schizophrenic deficit syndrome. Schizophr Bull 10:388–398, 1984

Leff J, Sartorius N, Jablensky A, et al: The International Pilot Study of Schizophrenia: five-year follow-up findings. Psychol Med 22:131–145, 1992

Loebel AD, Lieberman JA, Alvir JMJ, et al: Duration of psychosis and outcome in first-episode schizophrenia. Am J Psychiatry 149:1183–1188, 1992

Ram R, Bromet E, Eaton W, et al: The natural course of schizophrenia: a review of first-admission studies. Schizophr Bull 18:185–207, 1992

Robinson D, Woerner MG, Alvir JM, et al: Predictors of relapse following response from a first episode of schizophrenia or schizoaffective disorder. Arch Gen Psychiatry 56:342–247, 1999

Schwartz JE, Fennig S, Karant, M, et al: Congruence of diagnoses 2 years after a first-admission diagnosis of psychosis. Arch Gen Psychiatry 57:593–600, 2000

Spitzer RL, Williams J, Gibbon M, et al: The Structured Clinical Interview for DSM-III-R (SCID): history, rationale, and description. Arch Gen Psychiatry 49:624–629, 1992

Strakowski SM, Keck PE, McElroy SL, et al: Twelve-month outcome after a first hospitalization for affective psychosis. Arch Gen Psychiatry 55:49–55, 1998

Vetter P, Köller O: Clinical and psychosocial variables in different diagnostic groups: their interrelationships and value as predictors of course and outcome during a 14-year follow-up. Psychopathology 29:159–168, 1996

Woerner M, Manuzza S, Kane J: Anchoring the BPRS: an aid to improved reliability. Psychopharmacol Bull 24:112–124, 1988

Wyatt RJ, Damiani M, Henter I: First-episode schizophrenia: early intervention and medication discontinuation in the context of course and treatment. Br J Psychiatry 72(suppl 33):77–83, 1998

3

Investigating the Early Stages of Schizophrenia

The Hillside Prospective Study of First-Episode Schizophrenia

Jeffrey A. Lieberman, M.D.

The formal onset of schizophrenia usually occurs as an acute psychotic episode in adolescence or early adulthood, but there is reason to believe that the basis for schizophrenia long predates its formal onset and that the illness has a genetic component. Patients are generally not thought to be premorbidly ill, but there may be subtle manifestations of the illness in terms of slight decrements in cognitive, motor, and social functions. However, these features are not grossly apparent or clearly outside the range of individuals that do not go on to develop schizophrenia. The

This work was supported by National Institute of Mental Health grants (MH41646, MH00537, MH41960) and the Hillside Hospital Mental Health Clinical Research Center for the Study of Schizophrenia. Many individuals made important contributions to this study in various capacities including Jose Alvir, Dr.PH.; Manzar Ashtari, Ph.D.; Robert Bilder, Ph.D.; Bernhard Bogerts, M.D.; Michael Borenstein, Ph.D.; Miranda Chakos, M.D.; Gustave DeGreef, M.D.; Stephen Geisler, M.D.; Darlene Jody, M.D.; John Kane, M.D.; Amy Koreen, M.D.; Deborah Levy, Ph.D.; Anthony Loebel, M.D.; David Mayerhoff, M.D.; Sabina Meyer; Brian Sheitman, M.D.; Sally Szymanski, M.D.; Margaret Woerner, Ph.D.; and Huwei Wu.

formal onset of schizophrenia is usually preceded by nonspecific prodromal signs that can worsen into psychotic symptoms. When psychotic signs occur, patients are usually eventually brought into treatment. However, the period of time until that first professional contact and therapeutic intervention varies markedly and may last for months and even years. Almost all patients recover from their first psychotic episode. Although a small proportion experience few or no recurrences, the overwhelming majority go on to develop subsequent episodes. In the course of these relapses, they may not recover as well as after the initial or preceding episode, and they are left with persistent symptoms and associated functional impairment. A longer duration of illness and more numerous psychotic episodes are established negative prognostic factors (McGlashan 1988). In addition, the duration of psychosis before treatment has been consistently correlated negatively with outcomes, whether assessed as remission from the first episode, time to relapse, or long-term outcome (Crow et al. 1986; Loebel et al. 1992; May et al. 1981; Wyatt 1991). These findings suggest that in the early phase of the illness, superimposed on the neurodevelopmental diathesis, an active neurodegenerative process may be occurring during acute psychosis; if this degenerative component is not counteracted, the patient may suffer persistent morbidity and show a reduced response to therapy (Lieberman 1999).

Unfortunately, in the tertiary-care settings in which most psychiatric research is conducted, patients with good prognoses are rare and most treatment studies contain primarily chronic patients who have experienced multiple episodes of illness. These samples are likely to contain patients who are not fully responsive to treatment, not compliant with treatment, or both. Furthermore, because almost all patients with schizophrenia are treated with antipsychotic medications, multiepisode patients usually have taken antipsychotic agents for prolonged periods, and this may confound efforts to examine the neurobiologic manifestations of the disorder and associations between predictor variables and treatment response. Additionally, if schizophrenia involves a neurodegenerative process, treatment response may change over the course of the illness and data from multiepisode samples may not accurately reflect potential response in first-episode patients.

Differences in neuropathology between patients with first-episode and those with chronic schizophrenia have been identified; chronic patients show higher rates and greater severity of pathology in the medial-temporal region and the ventricular system (Bogerts et al. 1990, 1993; Lieberman et al. 1992, 1996b). However, the differences could be caused either by neuropathological progression during the early phase of the illness or by the fact that chronically ill patients are a more severely affected population who respond less well to treatment.

The best way to investigate the nature of clinical and pathophysiological progression of schizophrenia and the factors that influence outcome is through prospective studies of first-episode patients. First-episode samples are not subject to the potential biases of samples that contain chronically ill patients and thus may be more representative of the full spectrum of treatment response in schizophrenia. Furthermore, first-episode patients are more homogeneous with respect to the stage of illness and are unaffected by previous antipsychotic therapeutic interventions. By following the longitudinal course and treatment outcomes of patients from their first episode, it may be possible to identify specific clinical and biological factors that predict the course of illness in terms of the patients' capacity for recovery and development of treatment resistance and thus provide clear information on the degenerative process that is hypothesized to be occurring in the early phase of the disorder (Lieberman 1999).

Although there have been numerous longitudinal studies of schizophrenic patients, including first-episode patients (reviewed in McGlashan 1988 and Chatterjee and Lieberman 1999), before 1990 few studies had used comprehensive assessments of the different domains of morbidity of the illness, and even fewer had controlled the treatment of patients studied long term from their first episode. No studies combined comprehensive clinical assessments and controlled treatment with biological assessments of brain morphology and neurochemical activity. Thus, the Prospective Study of Psychobiology in First Episode Schizophrenia, conducted over a 10-year period at Hillside Hospital and described in this chapter, played a pivotal role in developing data on the characteristics, course, and treatment outcomes of first-episode patients and focused attention on the early stages of schizophrenia. This study prospectively followed patients from their first episodes and used concurrent assessments of clinical and biological variables to explore the course of schizophrenia and examine predictors of treatment response. A selective summary of the methods and results that have been previously published follows.

Description of Methods

Over a 10-year period, from 1986 through 1996, all patients admitted to the inpatient services of Hillside Hospital in Glen Oaks, New York, for their first episode of psychosis were examined for study eligibility. To be eligible, patients had to meet the Research Diagnostic Criteria (Spitzer et al. 1977) for a diagnosis of definite or probable schizophrenia or schizoaffective disorder, mainly schizophrenia, based on an interview using the Schedule for Affective Disorders and Schizophrenia (SADS; Spitzer and Endicott 1978). In addition, eligible patients had to have at least one current psychotic symptom (e.g., delusions, hallucinations, impaired understandability, derailment, illogical thinking or bizarre behavior) of sufficient severity to achieve a rating of 4 or more on the SADS Change Version with Psychosis and Disorganization Scale (SADS–C+PD; Spitzer and Endicott 1978). Eligible patients had experienced no prior psychotic episodes, had received fewer than 12 weeks of prior (lifetime) neuroleptic treatment, had no medical contraindications to treatment with antipsychotic medications, and had no history of neuromedical illness (e.g., endocrinopathy, hydrocephalus, seizure disorder) that could influence the diagnosis or the biological variables assessed in the study. Patients were between the ages of 16 and 40 years.

Patients who had received antipsychotic treatment immediately before hospital admission were maintained drug free for at least 14 days. Before initiation of treatment, baseline evaluations were conducted using the following assessments: the SADS–C+PD, Scale for the Assessment of Negative Symptoms (SANS; Andreasen 1983), Clinical Global Impressions (CGI) Scale (Guy 1976a), Simpson-Angus Neurologic Rating Scales (Simpson and Angus 1970), and Simpson Dyskinesia Scale (SDS; Simpson et al. 1979). Patients underwent challenge procedures with methylphenidate hydrochloride and apomorphine hydrocholoride, and baseline assessments of brain morphologic features on magnetic resonance imaging and smooth pursuit eye movements.

During their initial hospitalization, patients' premorbid status was investigated using the Premorbid Adjustment Scale (PAS; Cannon-Spoor et al. 1982), which assesses premorbid social and role functioning during childhood, early adolescence, late adolescence, and adulthood. Age at onset and mode of onset of illness were ascertained through interviews with patients and family members. Multiple informants were available and were used to obtain data for all study subjects. Onset of illness was determined first by asking patients and family members when the patient first experienced (or the family member noticed) behavioral changes that, in retrospect, appeared to have been related to the patient's becoming ill. Second, after explaining what psychosis is, we asked when the patient first experienced psychotic symptoms and when the family member first noticed such symptoms. When patient and family member responses differed, the research team reached a consensus decision. All evaluations were made by staff members who were blinded to patients' treatment response and outcomes. The methods of the study have been reported in more detail elsewhere (Lieberman et al. 1992, 1993a, 1993b; Robinson et al. 1999a, 1999b).

Treatment Protocol

After baseline evaluation procedures, patients were treated openly with traditional antipsychotic agents in accordance with a standard algorithm. The initial medication given was fluphenazine, 20 mg/day orally for 6 weeks. If the conditions of patients were not improved after 6 weeks, the fluphenazine dosage was doubled to 40 mg/day orally for an additional 4 weeks. If still unimproved, patients were switched to haloperidol, 20 mg/day orally for 6 weeks. If they were still unresponsive, the haloperidol dosage was increased to 40 mg/day for 4 more weeks. If patients remained unresponsive, a third antipsychotic from a different biochemical class, molindone (up to 300 mg/day) or loxapine (up to 150 mg/day) was attempted for up to 6 weeks. Adjunctive treatment with lithium was given at the end of either the haloperidol or the molindone trial. (Because of a protocol modification during the course of the study, not all eligible patients received the lithium augmentation.) Finally, treatment-resistant patients were treated with clozapine, up to 900 mg/day.

Fourteen patients in the study received some treatment that did not conform to the standard medication algorithm. Eleven started treatment with a typical antipsychotic agent other than fluphenazine in pilot versions of the protocol. Three patients began treatment with fluphenazine, but for a variety of clinical reasons, they subsequently received antipsychotic agents not specified in the algorithm.

Antiparkinsonian medication was not administered prophylactically so the incidence of acute extrapyramidal symptoms (EPS) could be determined. If acute EPS developed, patients were given benztropine mesylate, 2 to 6 mg/day. For patients with akathisia, lorazepam was used; if it was ineffective, propanolol was tried. Adjuvant medications for mood stabilization were used as clinically warranted. Patients who did not respond to the treatment algorithm were given additional medications as deemed clinically indicated by the research team.

Clinical Assessments

During the acute treatment phase, patients were evaluated for behavioral response and side effects biweekly for 12 weeks and thereafter every 4 weeks with the SADS–C+PD, SANS, CGI, and a modified Simpson-Angus

Extrapyramidal Scale (SAEPS). Evaluations with a modified SDS were completed every 8 weeks. The SDS includes 28 items with a 6-point global score ranging from 0 (no tardive dyskinesia [TD]) to 5 (severe TD). In addition, seven body area items that correspond to the Abnormal Involuntary Movement Scale (AIMS; Guy 1976b) were scored on a scale of 0–5.

Patients were considered to have shown improvement if they showed a decrease in psychopathologic features after 6 weeks to a point at which three of the four SADS–C+PD Positive Psychotic Symptom items were rated 3 (mild) or lower and the CGI Improvement rating was "much improved" or "very much improved." If patients showed continuing improvement or achieved remission, they continued to receive the initial treatment with fluphenazine. Patients were considered to have remitted when they had no rating greater than 3 on any of the SADS–C+PD Positive Psychotic Symptom items (i.e., suspiciousness, severity of delusions, severity of hallucinations, impaired understandability, bizarre behavior); a CGI Severity item rating of 3 (mild) or less; and a CGI Improvement item rating of 2 (much improved) or 1 (very much improved). This level of remission was required to persist for 8 weeks (four consecutive biweekly ratings). Sixteen weeks after they had met remission criteria, patients were rated on their level of remission in terms of whether they had residual symptoms (positive or negative). Patients were classified as fully remitted if they had no residual positive symptoms and no rating greater than 2 (mild) on the negative symptom global items of the SANS (e.g., affective flattening, alogia, attention), and they were considered partially remitted if they had persisting positive symptoms, though still below the levels required to meet remission criteria, or negative symptoms (SANS negative symptom global items above mild).

Patients who relapsed subsequent to the initial remission were treated with the same medication and dose to which they had first responded. If necessary, depending on clinical response, they then received further treatment according to the algorithm described previously.

When the study began, there was no limitation on length of participation. Later, the maximum length of participation was fixed at 5 years and patients who had been in the protocol longer than that were terminated. The longest period that a patient was followed without responding from the initial episode was 76 months.

Risk Factors

The following definitions were used for risk factors examined as predictors of treatment response: obstetric complications were considered present if the patient had one or more level 5 "potentially greatly harmful/relevant" events on the McNeil-Sjostrom Scale (McNeil et al. 1994); severity of baseline hallucinations and delusions was determined by the mean of the ratings on these items of the SADS–C+PD; severity of baseline disorganization was defined as the mean of the SADS–C+PD rating for bizarre behavior, inappropriate affect, and a composite measure of thought disorder consisting of the mean of the impaired understandability, derailment, and illogical thinking items; and severity of baseline negative symptoms was determined by the mean of the global ratings for affective flattening, alogia, avolition-apathy, and anhedonia-asociality of the SANS. The severity of baseline depressive symptoms was measured by a Hamilton Rating Scale for Depression (HRSD) score extracted from the SADS–C+PD. Baseline EPS were considered present if patients had a score of 1 (mild) or more on the items of rigidity, cogwheel rigidity, akinesia, or bradykinesia on the SAEPS. Parkinsonism was present if the patient had a rating of 3 (marked) or more on the rigidity item or a rating of 2 (moderate) on rigidity and 2 (definitely present) on the cogwheeling items of the SAEPS; akathisia was present if the patient had a rating of 2 (moderate) or greater on the akathisia SAEPS item. During treatment and follow-up, EPS was defined operationally as having at least two scores of 2 (mild) or one score of 3 (moderate) on any of the modified SAEPS items for gait, rigidity, tremor, akinesia, or akathisia or as having a "yes" response on the item for dystonia within the first episode of illness.

Patients who received a global score of 1 (questionable TD) or greater on the SDS, as rated by the research psychiatrist, were sent for rating confirmation by three designated expert raters, who were blinded to the patient's stage of illness and treatment. Patients who received a global TD rating of at least 2 (mild TD) on the SDS according to each of the three expert raters, independently, were considered to have presumptive TD. Patients who met criteria for presumptive TD and whose TD symptoms persisted for at least 3 months in follow-up evaluations by the expert raters were considered to have persistent TD. Interrater reliability was 0.91 on the SDS global items.

Biological Assessments

During the baseline period, patients underwent challenge procedures with methylphenidate and apomorphine (Lieberman et al. 1993a). These procedures were performed in a fixed order (apomorphine first) 72 hours apart, between 8 A.M. and 11 A.M. after an all-night fast. After the methylphenidate infusion, the patients' behavioral responses were rated on every behavioral item of the SADS–C+PD and the SANS. Growth hormone levels in response to apomorphine were assessed by serial collection of whole blood before and after apomorphine administration; specimens were analyzed by radioimmunoassay.

Plasma homovanillic acid (HVA) was examined at baseline by indwelling catheter serial sample collection and by weekly venipuncture during acute treatment under standardized conditions (Koreen et al. 1994a).

Magnetic resonance images of the brain were obtained at baseline, as soon after study entry as possible, and at approximately 18-month intervals during the follow-up period. Qualitative evaluations by visual inspection were performed under blind conditions by raters trained in neuroanatomy (Lieberman et al. 1992). Using operational criteria, a consensus determination was made as to the absence or presence of marked or mild abnormal morphology in each of four regions (i.e., lateral ventricles, third ventricle, frontal or parietal cortex, medial temporal cortex). Subjects with one or more areas classified as abnormal were termed globally abnormal. We also performed quantitative analyses of magnetic resonance images using a computer-based automated mensuration system to assess anatomically defined regions of interest (Ashtari et al. 1990; Bilder et al. 1994; Bogerts et al. 1990; DeGreef et al. 1992a, 1992b).

A total of 62 physically and psychologically healthy control subjects were recruited for comparative biological assessments through advertisements in the local media. Volunteers were screened for medical and psychiatric illness and drug abuse history and underwent a Structured Clinical Interview (SCID) and physical examination with laboratory testing. Eligible subjects were matched in age, gender, race, and socioeconomic status to study patients.

Statistical Methods

Survival analytic techniques were used to estimate the cumulative rate of treatment response and the effects of potential predictors of treatment response. These techniques were considered most appropriate for our data because the lengths of follow-up times differed for patients. In addition, not all patients responded to treatment during the follow-up period.

The effects of single and multiple potential predictors of response were analyzed using Cox proportional hazards regression. Because of the large number of predictors included in the analyses, we set statistical significance at $P<0.01$. We thus used 99% confidence intervals to indicate the precision of the hazard ratios.

Results

During this 10-year study, 807 patients were screened for eligibility. Of these, 410 did not meet the study criteria because of inappropriate diagnosis (n=320), medical contraindications (n=6), age (n=44), or previous treatment (n=33); an additional 7 patients were ruled ineligible for administrative reasons. Of the eligible 397 patients, 123 refused to participate and 94 were excluded for clinical or administrative reasons (e.g., involuntary status, history of extreme violence). Thus, 180 eligible patients (45%) consented to participate and entered the study. A total of 36 patients were later withdrawn because of a change in diagnosis based on additional information (n=20), discovery of severe substance abuse history (n=4), magnetic resonance imaging findings indicative of neurologic illness (n=4), discovery of prior antipsychotic treatment (n=1), or administrative reasons (n=7). Of the remaining 144 patients, 26 patients who entered the study in the later years and were treated with either risperidone or clozapine to examine the effects of atypical antipsychotic drugs on first-episode patients were excluded from the analyses. Thus, 118 patients are included in this report.

The demographic characteristics of patients who did and did not enter the study did not differ significantly. Thus the study patients were considered representative of the overall population of patients with first-episode schizophrenia.

The sample of 118 patients was 52% male; had a mean age of 25.2 years; and was 42% Caucasian, 37% African American, 12% Hispanic, 7% Asian, and 3% mixed racial or ethnic background. Thus, the sample included significant representation of female subjects and the major racial and ethnic groups in the area. There was a range of socioeconomic classes and educational levels, but patients were predominantly middle class and below (mean socioeconomic status on the Hollingshead Redlich Scale was 3.4).

Patients had been ill for an extended period; the mean time since the first appearance of behavioral changes related to the illness was 143 weeks, and the mean time since exhibiting formal psychotic symptoms was 71 weeks. It was surprising that many patients had had active psychotic symptoms for so long before coming to treatment. This suggests a general failure to bring psychotic patients into the health care system early. However, we do not know the cause of this; patients or their families may have failed to seek care, care may not have been easily available, or it is possible that patients were not immediately diagnosed.

At study entry, the patients were severely ill, with a mean CGI score of 5.5 and a mean Global Assessment of Functioning (GAS; Endicott et al. 1976) score of 27.1. Based on Research Diagnostic Criteria, 83 were diagnosed with schizophrenia (53% paranoid, 11% undifferentiated, 4% disorganized, 2% catatonic subtypes), and 35 were diagnosed with schizoaffective disorder. Using Research Diagnostic Criteria, 21% were acute, 36% subacute, 14% subchronic, and 29% chronic. A total of 73% had received no antipsychotic agents before admission; 16% had taken less than 2 weeks of medication; and 11% had had between 2 and 12 weeks of exposure. Interestingly, poor global adjustment status in childhood and early and late adolescence as measured by the Premorbid Adjustment Scale was associated with earlier age of illness onset, longer duration of psychiatric and psychotic symptoms, and poorer treatment response and outcome (Strous et al. in press). This suggests that the onset of illness may long precede the appearance of psychotic symptoms by which a formal diagnosis can be made.

The cumulative percentage of patients remitting by 52 weeks was 87% (95% CI, 80.4%, 93.1%); the median time to recovery was 9 weeks (95% CI, 8%, 12%). When patients were rated in terms of their level of recovery from the first episode of illness, 73% were fully remitted (i.e., no persisting symptoms and return to premorbid level of function), 16% were partially remitted (i.e., mild residual positive symptoms or moderate residual negative symptoms), and 11% were nonremitted (i.e., persisting positive symptoms of moderate severity or greater) (Robinson et al. 1999b). Global outcomes were rated at 6 months after patients fulfilled remission criteria, based on treatment response, presence of residual symptoms, extent of recovery to premorbid status, and global level of function. Outcomes for 22% of the patients were rated excellent, 40% good, 28% fair, and 10% poor (treatment-refractory patients). Thus, more than two thirds of the sample had a good outcome from their first episode of illness.

The mean antipsychotic dosage in fluphenazine equivalents while the patients were in the first acute treatment period was 18.9 (SD, 8.7) mg/day. Neither antipsychotic drug dosage nor drug level predicted treatment outcome in Cox analyses in which dosage was a time-varying covariate ($\chi^2=0.11$, $df=1$, $P=0.75$)(Koreen et al. 1994b; Robinson et al. 1999b). However, this analysis was constrained by the fact that patients were treated with a standardized protocol that allowed little variability in dose.

To obtain a fuller view of patients whose illnesses were refractory to treatment of the first episode, we reviewed the records of the 10 patients who failed to meet response criteria despite being treated for 1 year or longer (Szymanski et al. 1994). All were diagnosed with schizophrenia (three paranoid, four undifferentiated, one disorganized, and one catatonic subtype). Although 48% of the patient sample was female, only two of the refractory patients were women. These patients were followed for 12–76 months and had persistent severe positive symptoms throughout. Seven of the 10 had a trial of clozapine. Clozapine was discontinued in three because of nonresponse and was continued in four patients long term; these four were able to remain in the community despite continued positive symptoms. Two patients also received electroconvulsive therapy, and two were eventually placed in state hospital facilities.

The protocol maintained patients on medication for the first year. During this period, the relapse rate was low (16%). After 1 year, patients were given the option of discontinuing medication if they were clinically stable; most elected to stop. A survival analysis with medication status as a time-dependent covariate indicated that the risk of relapse was five times greater for those not taking medication than those taking medication.

The cumulative relapse rate for the 104 patients who successfully recovered from the first episode was 81.9% (95% CI, 70.6%–93.2%) at 5 years; for the 63 patients who recovered from their second episode, the cumulative relapse rate at 5 years was 78% (95% CI, 46.5%–100%); for the 20 patients who recovered from their third episode, the cumulative relapse rate at 4 years was 86% (95% CI, 61.5%–100%) (Robinson et al. 1999a). Thus, even for patients who fully recover, there is a high risk of relapse, particularly when they are not taking medication.

To examine the consistency of treatment response across episodes, time to response of patients who were similarly treated was analyzed. The mean times to remission for patients who had two episodes were 71 days (SD, 63) for the first and 78 (SD, 101) for the second episode. The mean times to remission for patients who had three episodes were 51 days ($n=36$), 62 days ($n=34$), and 104 days ($n=18$), respectively (Lieberman et al. 1996b). Although many factors can influence patients' treatment response and vulnerability to relapse, our findings show a pattern of decreasing responsiveness to treatment over subsequent episodes of illness. This could be because of the progression of the disease at the pathophysiological level as well as the psychopathological level or to the effects of treatment (e.g., through the development of tolerance to the therapeutic effects of antipsychotic drugs or from their toxicity). Whatever the cause, these results suggest that there are at least two forms of treatment resistance. The first is the form in which patients are treatment resistant in their first episode. We speculate that this type may be caused by neurodevelopmental pathology that is nonreversible. The second is manifested in patients who initially are responsive to treatment but become progressively less responsive to treatment in the context of recurrent episodes (Lieberman et al. 1998; Sheitman and Lieberman 1998).

Predictors of Treatment Response

Diagnosis (i.e., of schizophrenia vs. schizoaffective disorder), baseline disorganization, negative symptoms, akathisia, and dystonia during the first 16 weeks of treatment, psychotic symptom activation in response to methylphenidate, and baseline motor function on neuropsychological testing were not related to treatment response.

Women were more likely to respond to treatment than were men (Szymanski et al. 1995). The specific effects of gender were examined in 54 patients: 29 men and 25 women. They did not differ significantly in their childhood, adolescent, or adulthood adjustment, but female patients were significantly older at the onset of psychotic symptoms (men, 21 years, SD 5; women, 24 years, SD 6). At baseline, female patients showed significantly less illogical thinking but more anxiety, inappropriate affect, and bizarre behavior than the men.

Patients with higher premorbid functioning in childhood and adolescence, more acute onset and shorter duration of illness, lower baseline severity of positive and negative symptoms, nondeficit state status, and absence of parkinsonian signs during antipsychotic drug treatment had significantly better treatment outcomes (Chakos et al. 1996; Mayerhoff et al. 1994; Strous et al. in press). Patients with more severe hallucinations and delusions and those with poorer attention at initial presentation were less likely to respond (Robinson et al. 1999b). Patients who developed parkinsonism during treatment were approximately half as likely to respond as patients without these signs (Chakos et al. 1996).

Patients had substantial psychopathology at baseline, including both positive and negative symptoms. The association between baseline symptom severity and treatment response was primarily accounted for by positive symptoms. When we classified patients according to criteria for the deficit state, adapted from Carpenter et al. (1988), we found no significant relationship between deficit state and treatment outcome when patients were required to have been remitted for at least 6 months and meet the full set of criteria (Mayerhoff et al. 1994). However, when the entire sample was included in the analysis, patients with the deficit or questionable deficit state had a poorer treatment response and outcome (Mantel Haenszel χ^2=5.3, df=1, P=0.02). Patients with the deficit state were also more likely to develop TD (Mantel-Cops χ^2=16.8; P=0.0001).

Among the 70 patients in whom depression was followed over time, depressive symptoms were very prevalent at the baseline evaluation (Koreen et al. 1993). Using liberal criteria (i.e., extracted HRSD scores of 15 or greater, Research Diagnostic Criteria depressive symptoms, or both), 75% were depressed. Most of the depressive symptoms occurred concurrently with psychotic symptoms and resolved as the psychosis remitted. However, depressive symptoms were not prodromal to a psychotic relapse and were not predictive of global outcome, time to reach remission, or a later postpsychotic depression. These findings are consistent with the view that depression is a core part of schizophrenia, at least early in the course of the illness.

One of the 118 patients had involuntary movements before treatment (Chatterjee et al. 1995). Nineteen patients developed presumptive TD during the study. Seventeen of these patients received global severity ratings of mild TD at the time of confirmation, and two received ratings of moderate TD. All 19 patients had body area global ratings of at least 2 in an orofacial region, and 11 had ratings of at least 2 in both orofacial and extremity or trunk regions. Ten patients met the criteria for persistent TD. Survival analysis indicated that the cumulative incidence of presumptive TD was 6.3% after 1 year of follow-up, 11.5% after 2 years, 13.7% after 3 years, and 17.5% after 4 years. The cumulative incidence of persistent TD was 4.8% after 1 year, 7.2% after 2 years, and 15.6% after 4 years. Antipsychotic drug treatment and treatment outcome were associated with TD development. Controlling for clozapine treatment, each 100-mg chlorpromazine equivalent increase in antipsychotic drug dose resulted in a 6% increase in the hazard of presumptive TD (hazard ratio, 1.06). Controlling for time to treatment response, responders had a significantly lower hazard for presumptive TD (hazard ratio, 0.07). The effects of treatment response and antipsychotic drug dose on persistent TD were similar to those for presumptive TD. TD was also related to greater impairment on the childhood PAS score, but when dose, clozapine exposure, treatment response, and time to response were controlled for, childhood PAS score was not a significant predictor of TD. These findings suggest that patients who are more severely ill and less responsive to treatment are more vulnerable to TD.

Interestingly, 17% of the drug-naïve sample had mild or moderate signs of EPS at baseline (Chatterjee et al. 1995). Patients with idiopathic EPS had higher levels of negative symptoms at baseline (3.1 vs. 2.4; $t = -2.6$, $df=790$, $P=0.01$), and they had a poorer treatment outcome in time to and level of remission ($\chi^2=7.9$, $df=2$, $P=0.02$).

Histories of obstetric complications were obtained for 59 of the patients (Alvir et al. 1999). Twelve of these 59 had positive histories of such complications, including four instances of prolonged labor; two instances each of emergency cesarean section, early bleeding, and less than 33 weeks' gestation; and one instance each of maternal smoking of two packs of cigarettes a day and syphilis, both during the third trimester. The child of one mother who underwent an emergency cesarean section also experienced fetal distress and exhibited meconium staining. One mother who underwent prolonged labor had attempted an abortion in the first trimester. The median time to treatment response was 11 weeks (95% CI, 8, 15) in the group of patients without obstetric complications and 39 weeks (95% CI, 28, 195) in the group with obstetric complications. Six patients, three in each group, had not responded to treatment at the last observation point. Cox proportional hazards regression analysis showed that patients in the group with positive history of obstetric complications were almost four times less likely to respond to treatment than those with negative histories (hazard ratio controlling for gender=0.28; 95% CI, 0.13, 0.62). There was no clear pattern of contribution of specific complications. Obstetric complications may reflect a neurobiological insult that contributes to the potential severity of a patient's illness, either independently or additively with other factors (e.g., genetic factors). This effect on illness severity may be only partially expressed by overt indices of illness severity but may significantly influence the capacity for treatment response. Thus, pathological disruption of neural circuits in a system that may already be dysfunctional from prior etiologic effects may increase the potential severity of illness and compromise the patient's capacity for treatment response and recovery.

To examine whether our predictor variables had independent or shared effects on treatment outcome, we performed a multivariate analysis using gender, baseline hallucinations, and delusions and parkinsonism as predictors (obstetric complications were not included in the analysis because data were available on too few patients). The analysis was run using data from 88 patients who had complete information on all three predictors. The hazard ratios were 1.79 (99% CI, 0.99, 3.25) for gender, 0.65 (99% CI, 0.47, 0.89) for baseline hallucinations and delusions, and 0.54 (99% CI, 0.22, 1.36) for parkinsonism.

Neuropsychological and Psychophysiological Characteristics

A total of 94 patients completed at least one comprehensive neuropsychological examination after stabilization of the first episode of schizophrenia or schizoaffective disorder (Bilder et al. 2000). The modal time from beginning of treatment to neuropsychological examination was 0.47 years (median, 0.61 years). Compared with the 62 control subjects, the patient group was more impaired on every neuropsychological dimension measured. Mean effect sizes ranged from −1.11 to −1.75; 95% CIs ranged from a minimum deficit of −0.82 to a maximum deficit of −2.13. The memory and executive scales showed significantly more impairment and the language scale less impairment than the remaining scales. More importantly, the overall profile mean for the patients was −1.53, indicating a generalized deficit of approximately 1.5 SD. This profile suggests a relatively nonspecific deficit pattern, which could reflect either diffuse dysfunction or disturbances in key systems that have modulatory effects on broadly distributed neural networks. Neuropsychological performance was not correlated with symptoms at study entry, but it was correlated with symptoms after clinical stabilization: patients with more severe, treatment-refractory symptoms had more neuropsychological impairment.

Normality of eye tracking was tested quantitatively and qualitatively by independent raters in 43 patients and 42 normal control subjects (Levy et al. 2000; Lieberman et al. 1993a). Neither the discriminant or composite score nor any of the individual quantitative measures significantly distinguished the eye tracking of schizophrenics from the eye tracking of the control subjects, although differences were always in the expected direction. The schizophrenic patients, however, had a significantly higher rate of qualitatively impaired eye tracking (21 of 43, or 48.8%) than the controls (2 of 42, or 4.8%). Furthermore, the schizophrenic patients with qualitatively impaired eye tracking had significantly higher discriminant scores than schizophrenic patients with normal eye tracking or normal control subjects. The heterogeneity in scores among the group of schizophrenic patients could not be explained by differences in symptom severity, hospitalization, age, gender, or duration of illness.

Indices of Dopamine Neural Activity

A total of 67 patients completed challenge tests with methylphenidate and apomorphine at baseline to measure central nervous system (CNS)

dopamine activity (Lieberman et al. 1993a). In response to methylphenidate, 59% of the patients exhibited symptom activation. Methylphenidate
nonactivators were more severely ill and had more positive and negative
symptoms than activators at baseline. Twenty-one of the patients tested
at baseline were retested after 6 months of remission and after a 2-week
drug washout. The activation rate was 29% compared with the 59% rate
at baseline. All patients who activated after remission had been activators
at baseline.

Baseline data on basal growth hormone levels in response to apomorphine challenge were available for 42 patients and 11 control subjects. Controlling for gender, patients with schizophrenia had significantly
higher mean basal growth hormone levels than control subjects ($t=2.7$,
$P=0.01$). Patients with higher mean basal growth hormone levels took
longer to remit (hazard ratio=0.94, 95% CI, 0.99, 1.02) and had poorer
outcomes (Mantel-Haenszel $\chi^2=3.4$, $df=1$, $P=0.07$).

It has been suggested that plasma HVA concentrations may reflect
brain dopamine activity, making this a useful tool for studying the pathophysiology of schizophrenia. In our study, baseline plasma HVA did not
differ between patients and control subjects and was not correlated with
baseline psychopathology; however, it was associated with residual negative symptoms after remission ($r=0.31$, $P<0.05$). Plasma HVA was significantly increased over baseline for the first 3 weeks of treatment and
subsequently declined to—but not below—baseline levels. However, patients were tested after only 6 weeks, which may not be long enough to
detect continued decrease. Baseline HVA predicted time to remission,
with those having higher levels responding sooner (hazard ratio 1.06;
95% CI, 1.002, 1.13). Women had significantly higher levels than men and
had a greater short-term increase with treatment.

Magnetic Resonance Imaging

Brain magnetic resonance images were obtained from 109 patients (51%
men) and 62 control subjects (52% men). Patients were qualitatively rated
as more abnormal than the control group ($\chi^2=7.3$, $df=2$, $P=0.02$) (Lieberman et al. 1993a). A total of 13% of the patients were rated as markedly
abnormal and 51% as mildly abnormal, with only 36% rated normal. In
contrast, 3% of the control subjects were markedly abnormal, 44% mildly
abnormal, and 53% normal. The highest prevalence of pathomorphology
was in the lateral ventricles, followed (in descending order of frequency)
by the third ventricle, medial temporal cortex, and frontal parietal occipital cortex. These data point to the relatively subtle nature of the neuro-

pathology of first-episode schizophrenia and the substantial variation in normal human neuroanatomy that overlaps with the neuropathology of schizophrenia. We also performed quantitative analyses of magnetic resonance images using a computer-based automated mensuration system. Comparison of the schizophrenia and control groups, controlling for age, gender, and height, revealed differences in total cortical (F=7.2, P=0.009) and ventricular volumes (F=2.9, P=0.09) (DeGreef et al. 1992b). The volume differences were relatively small: 3% for the cortex and 17% for the ventricles (an absolute difference of only 2.8 mL). The fact that differences were small reflects the subtle nature of the neuropathology of schizophrenia noted previously and may reflect the likelihood that neuropathology is not fully manifest in patients with first-episode schizophrenia; rather, it is progressive over the illness.

Comparison of medial temporal cortex volumes revealed similar differences between patients with schizophrenia and control patients (Bogerts et al. 1990). Hippocampal volume was smaller (19%) in schizophrenic patients than it was in control subjects. Volume differences in the anterior and posterior sections bilaterally ranged from 6% to 24%. The volume differences were greater in men and on the left side, but there were no significant group-by-gender or group-by-hemisphere interactions.

Healthy control subjects showed systematic asymmetries of cerebral hemispheric volume. The prefrontal, premotor, and temporal regions were larger on the right side, and the sensorimotor and occipitoparietal regions were larger on the left. Patients did not show this pattern; they had less absolute asymmetry in all regions and significantly less asymmetry in the occipitoparietal, premotor, and prefrontal regions. Patients with the undifferentiated subtype of schizophrenia at the time of diagnosis had less asymmetry than did those diagnosed with the paranoid subtype; among men, less normal asymmetry was correlated with higher ratings of negative symptoms.

An unexpected finding was a strikingly high rate of noncommunicating (i.e., nontraumatic) cavum septum pellucidum in patients (DeGreef et al. 1992a). Sixteen of the 109 patients evaluated were found to have a cavum septum, compared with 4 of the 62 control subjects. This suggests a failure in normal neuroanatomical maturation in these patients.

In this study, we found no difference in caudate nuclei volume between patients and control subjects. Because this differs from findings previously reported for chronic patients, we conducted a follow-up analysis of caudate nucleus volumes and found a surprising increase after treatment with typical antipsychotic agents (Chakos et al. 1994). The increase may have been the result of an interaction between neuroleptic treatment and the plasticity of dopaminergic neuronal systems in young patients. The increase was reversed after treatment with the atypical antipsychotic agent clozapine (Chakos et al. 1994, 1995).

It appears that brain pathomorphology is associated with disease severity, male gender, earlier age of onset, more primary negative symptoms, greater likelihood of developing the deficit state, longer time to remission, and poorer outcome.

Conclusions

In general, patients in their first episode of schizophrenia respond to antipsychotic drug treatment very well and have good prognoses. Almost all our patients (87%) recovered or achieved substantial symptom remission within 1 year, and the median time to response was only 9 weeks. The response rate is remarkable when compared with the response rates reported for multiepisode patients, especially because our response criteria were more stringent than those often used in treatment studies. Although our overall response rate was very high, 10 patients were refractory to intensive treatment efforts, including clozapine. It is clear that studies of other second-generation antipsychotic or treatment agents are needed for patients such as these.

However, despite the high level of recovery from their first episode, the vast majority of patients experienced recurrences of their illness in the form of psychotic relapses within the 5-year period of follow-up. This should cause us to reconsider the current guidelines for the appropriate length of follow-up treatment for first-episode patients.

The high rate of recurrence, increasing length of time, and decreasing proportion of patients achieving symptom remission over subsequent psychotic episodes reflected, we believe, the progression of the illness. We have recently presented longitudinal neuroimaging data that appear to support this interpretation (Lieberman et al. 2001).

Several significant relationships between baseline demographic and clinical variables and treatment response emerged from our analyses. Women were more likely to respond than men. Patients with more severe positive symptoms and worse attention at study entry were less likely to respond. Patients with a history of obstetric complications were almost four times less likely to respond than patients without such a history. Patients with enlarged lateral ventricles responded less well to treatment.

Patients with spontaneous EPS before treatment and patients who later developed TD or parkinsonism were also less likely to respond. However, our algorithm used higher medication doses than are often now used in first-episode patients. The algorithm also emphasized conventional agents, with clozapine for patients who were resistant to conventional agents. This medication strategy probably produced more motor side effects than a lower-dose conventional antipsychotic or first-line novel agent would produce.

Clearly, the patients participating in multiepisode studies do not include those who respond best to initial treatment. Nevertheless, given the very high rate of response of these first-episode patients to treatment, an obvious question is why multiepisode patients in most studies respond so poorly. It is possible, of course, that the difference in treatment response between first-episode and chronic multiepisode patients may be explained by the patient selection process. Our hypothesis, however, is that the pathophysiological processes in schizophrenia unfold in three stages over the life of the patient and correspond to specific phases of the illness. To summarize, we suggest that the initial developmental insult to the CNS (stage 1) does not result in psychosis until a combination of developmental and dysregulatory events occur, causing sensitization (stage 2), which then can lead to the formal onset of illness. If persistent or recurrent, the illness episodes can progress to a self-limiting degenerative phase (stage 3) manifested by persistent morbidity, treatment resistance, and clinical deterioration (Lieberman 1999; Lieberman et al. 1997).

This hypothesis suggests that longer duration of psychoses is associated with poorer treatment response and higher levels of residual symptoms and morbidity. Furthermore, patients exhibit greater sensitivity to stress and psychostimulants in the earlier phases of the illness. More severe forms of psychopathology are associated with longer duration of psychoses and occur in later stages of the illness. Antipsychotic treatment resistance develops over the course of the illness and is most prevalent in the later stages.

These remain hypotheses and, therefore, are tentative. The predictions need to be tested in additional studies and with new samples. In the meantime, given what we now know, treatment interventions that limit the duration and number of psychotic episodes, particularly with second-generation agents, should prevent the development of treatment resistance, severe forms of psychopathology, and progression of brain neuropathology and reduce the likelihood of TD (Lieberman et al. 1996b). Thus, the optimal principles for treating patients with schizophrenia and preventing treatment resistance appear to be early identification and intervention with psychotic patients; effective treatment with maximal effort to prevent relapse, including the minimization of noxious side effects that may lead to noncompliance; use of the lowest effective dose; and early use of clozapine therapy at the first indication that a patient may be developing treatment resistance.

This study, which was conducted over a 10-year period, has produced a number of findings and contributed to the development of pathophysiological hypotheses. It has also served to focus the attention of the field on the early stages of schizophrenia, which has emerged as a key phase in the natural history of the illness in which to investigate its clinical phenomenology and pathophysiology and target treatment interventions. The latter consequence has provided impetus for the early identification and intervention strategy in the prodromal phase of schizophrenia, which has captured the field's imagination because of the prospect of preventing the onset of the disorder (Lieberman and Fenton 2000). Indeed, to understand and treat patients with the disorder we call schizophrenia, we seem, increasingly, to be starting with the disorder and working backwards.

References

Alvir JMJ, Woerner MG, Gunduz H, et al: Obstetric complications predict treatment response in first episode schizophrenia. Psychol Med 29: 621–627, 1999

Andreasen NC: The Scale for the Assessment of Negative Symptoms (SANS). Iowa City, IA, University of Iowa, 1983

Ashtari M, Zito JL, Gold B, et al: Computerized volume mensuration of brain structure. J Invest Radiol 27:798–805, 1990

Bilder RM, Wu H, Bogerts B, et al: Absence of regional hemispheric volume asymmetries in first episode schizophrenia. Am J Psychiatry 151:1437–1447, 1994

Bilder RM, Goldman RS, Robinson D, et al: Neuropsychology of first-episode schizophrenia: initial characterization and clinical correlates. Am J Psychiatry 157:549–559, 2000

Bogerts B, Ashtari M, Degreef G, et al: Reduced temporal limbic structure volumes on magnetic resonance images in first-episode schizophrenia. Psychiatry Res 35:1–3, 1990

Bogerts B, Lieberman JA, Ashtari M, et al: Hippocampus-amygdala volumes and psychopathology in chronic schizophrenia. Biol Psychiatry 33:236–246, 1993

Cannon-Spoor HE, Potkin SG, Wyatt RJ: Measurement of premorbid adjustment in chronic schizophrenia. Schizophr Bull 8:471–484, 1982

Carpenter WT, Heinrichs DW, Wagman AMI: Deficit and non-deficit forms of schizophrenia: the concept. Am J Psychiatry 145: 578–583, 1988

Chakos MH, Lieberman JA, Bilder RM, et al: Increase in caudate nuclei volumes of first episode schizophrenic patients taking antipsychotic drugs. Am J Psychiatry 151:1430–1436, 1994

Chakos MH, Lieberman JA, Alvir J, et al: Caudate nuclei volumes in schizophrenic patients treated with typical antipsychotics or clozapine. Lancet 345:456, 1995

Chakos MH, Alvir JMJ, Woerner MG, et al: Incidence and correlates of tardive dyskinesia in first episode of schizophrenia. Arch Gen Psychiatry 53:313–319, 1996

Chatterjee A, Lieberman JA: Studies of first-episode schizophrenia: a comprehensive review, in The Recognition and Management of Early Psychosis: A Preventive Approach. Edited by Jackson HJ, McGorry P, Perris C. Cambridge, United Kingdom, Cambridge University Press, 1999, pp 115–154

Chatterjee A, Chakos M, Koreen A, et al: Prevalence and clinical correlates of extrapyramidal signs and spontaneous dyskinesias in never medicated schizophrenic patients. Am J Psychiatry 152:1724–1729, 1995

Crow TJ, MacMillan JF, Johnson AL, et al: A randomised controlled trial of prophylactic neuroleptic treatment. Br J Psychiatry 428:120–127, 1986

Degreef G, Bogerts B, Falkai P, et al: Increased prevalence of the cavum septum pellucidum in MRI scans and post mortem brains of schizophrenic patients. Psychiatry Research: Neuroimaging 45:1–13, 1992a

Degreef G, Ashtari M, Bogerts B, et al: Volumes of ventricular system subdivisions measured from magnetic resonance images in first-episode schizophrenic patients. Arch Gen Psychiatry 49:531–537, 1992b

Guy W: Abnormal involuntary movement scale, in ECDEU Assessment Manual for Psychopharmacology. Washington, DC, U.S. Public Health Service, 1976a, pp 534–537

Guy W: Clinical global impression scale, in EDCEU Assessment Manual for Psychopharmacology. Washington, DC, U.S. Public Health Service, 1976b, pp 218–222

Koreen A, Siris SG, Chakos M, et al: Depression in first episode schizophrenia. Am J Psychiatry 150:1643–1648, 1993

Koreen A, Lieberman JA, Alvir J, et al: Plasma homovanillic acid in first episode schizophrenia: Psychopathology and treatment response. Arch Gen Psychiatry 51:132–138, 1994a

Koreen A, Lieberman JA, Alvir J, et al: Relation of plasma fluphenazine levels to treatment response and extrapyramidal side effects in first episode schizophrenic patients. Am J Psychiatry 151:35–39, 1994b

Levy DL, Lajonchere CM, Dorogusker B, et al: Quantative characterization of eye tracking dysfunction in schizophrenia. Schizophr Res 42:171–185, 2000

Lieberman JA: Atypical antipsychotic drugs as a first-line treatment of schizophrenia: a rationale and hypothesis. J Clin Psychiatry 57(suppl 11):68–71, 1996

Lieberman JA: Is schizophrenia a neurodegenerative disorder? a clinical and neurobiological perspective. Biol Psychiatry 46:729–739, 1999

Lieberman JA, Fenton WS: Delayed detection of psychosis: causes, consequences, and effect on public health. Am J Psychiatry 157:1727–1734, 2000

Lieberman JA, Alvir JMJ, Woerner M, et al: Prospective study of psychobiology in first episode schizophrenia at Hillside Hospital: design, methodology and summary of findings. Schizophr Bull 18:351–371, 1992

Lieberman JA, Jody D, Alvir JMJ, et al: Brain morphology, dopamine and eye tracking abnormalities in first-episode schizophrenia: prevalence and clinical correlates. Arch Gen Psychiatry 50:357–368, 1993a

Lieberman JA, Jody D, Geisler S, et al: Time course and biologic correlates of treatment response in first episode schizophrenia. Arch Gen Psychiatry 50:369–376, 1993b

Lieberman JA, Koreen AR, Chakos M, et al: Factors influencing treatment response and outcome of first-episode schizophrenia: implications for understanding the pathphysiology of schizophrenia. J Clin Psychiatry 57(suppl 9):5–9, 1996a

Lieberman JA, Alvir JM, Koreen A, et al: Psychobiologic correlates of treatment response in schizophrenia. Neuropsychopharmacology 14(suppl S):13–21, 1996b

Lieberman JA, Sheitman B, Kinon BJ: Neurochemical sensitization in the pathophysiology of schizophrenia: deficits and dysfunction in neuronal regulation and plasticity. Neuropsychopharmacology 17:205–229, 1997

Lieberman JA, Sheitman B, Chakos M, et al: The development of treatment resistance in patients with schizophrenia: a clinical and pathophysiological perspective. J Clin Psychopharmacol 18(suppl 1):20–24, 1998

Lieberman JA, Chakos M, Wu H, et al: Longitudinal study of brain morphology in first episode schizophrenia. Biol Psychiatry 49:487–499, 2001

Loebel AD, Lieberman JA, Alvir JMJ, et al: Duration of psychosis and outcome in first episode schizophrenia. Am J Psychiatry 149:1183–1188, 1992

May PR, Tuma AH, Dixon WJ: Schizophrenia: a follow-up study of the results of the five forms of treatment. Arch Gen Psychiatry 38:776–784, 1981

Mayerhoff DI, Loebel AD, Borenstein M, et al: The deficit state in first-episode schizophrenia. Am J Psychiatry 151:1417–1422, 1994

McGlashan TH: A selective review of recent North American long-term follow-up studies of schizophrenia. Schizophr Bull 14:515–542, 1988

McNeil TF, Cantor-Graae E, Sjostrom K: Obstetric complications as antecedents of schizophrenia: empirical effects of using different obstetric complication scales. J Psychiatr Res 28:519–530, 1994

Robinson D, Woerner M, Alvir J, et al: Predictors of relapse following response from a first episode of schizophrenia or schizoaffective disorder. Arch Gen Psychiatry 56:241–247, 1999a

Robinson D, Woerner M, Alvir J, et al: Predictors of treatment response from a first episode of schizophrenia or schizoaffective disorder. Am J Psychiatry 156:544–549, 1999b

Sheitman BB, Lieberman JA: The natural history and pathophysiology of treatment resistant schizophrenia. J Psychiatr Res 32:143–150, 1998

Simpson FM, Angus JWS: A rating scale for extrapyramidal side-effects. Acta Psychiatr Scand 212(suppl):11–19, 1970

Simpson GM, Lee JH, Zoubek B, et al: A rating scale for tardive dyskinesia. Psychopharmacology 64:171–179, 1979

Spitzer RL, Endicott J: Schedule for Affective Disorders and Psychosis and Disorganization Change Version, 3rd Edition. New York, Biometrics Research Division, New York State Psychiatric Institute, 1978

Spitzer RL, Endicott J, Robins E: Research Diagnostic Criteria for a Selected Group of Functional Disorders, 3rd Edition. New York, Biometrics Resarch Division, New York State Psychiatric Institute, 1977

Strous RD, Alvir JMJ, Robertson D, et al: Premorbid function in schizophrenia: relation to baseline symptoms, treatment response, and medication side effects. Schizophr Bull, in press

Szymanski S, Masiar S, Mayerhoff D, et al: Clozapine response in treatment-refractory first episode schizophrenia. Biol Psychiatry 35:278–280, 1994

Szymanski S, Lieberman JA, Alvir JM, et al: Gender differences in onset of illness, treatment response, course, and biologic indexes in first-episode schizophrenic patients. Am J Psychiatry 152:698–703, 1995

Wyatt RJ: Neuroleptics and the natural course of schizophrenia. Schizophr Bull 17:325–351, 1991

PART II

Management of the Early Stages of Schizophrenia

4

Optimal Pharmacologic Management of the First Episode of Schizophrenia

Robert B. Zipursky, M.D.

T reatment with antipsychotic medication is the foundation necessary for achieving recovery from a first episode of psychosis. Furthermore, the degree to which pharmacotherapy is successful likely defines the potential for long-term recovery. Treatment of the first episode represents a critical opportunity to intervene in a way that will bring about the greatest degree of remission at an early stage of the illness. Although the potential for positively affecting a patient's outcome is enormous at this stage of illness, so is the potential for doing great harm. The degree of the patient's engagement with treatment is often highly tenuous at this stage; if medication is prescribed in a way that results in frightening and uncomfortable side effects, the patient's willingness to receive treat-

The studies summarized in this chapter represent the combined work of many colleagues in our First Episode Psychosis and PET Programs, including Shitij Kapur, Gary Remington, and Jaihui Zhang-Wong. I would also like to express my gratitude to our study participants and their families for their involvement in our research studies. This research has been supported by the Canadian Institutes of Health Research, the National Alliance for Research on Schizophrenia and Affective Disorders, and the National Health Research and Development Program of Canada.

ment may be compromised in both the short and long term.

It is not uncommon to see untreated chronically ill patients who describe the traumatic experience of receiving antipsychotic medications for the first time and decide that they will never accept medication again. Adverse side effects may well result in refusal of any further treatment, and the opportunity to intervene at the critical early stage of the illness may be completely lost. The recent focus on early intervention has allowed several centers to develop extensive experience in working with this group of patients and to study the most efficacious means of prescribing antipsychotic medication to this group. This chapter reviews recent treatment studies and provides a framework for the optimal use of antipsychotic medications in the treatment of patients with a first episode of schizophrenia.

What Are the Objectives of Treatment?

To evaluate the success of antipsychotic treatment, it is imperative that the objectives of pharmacotherapy be clear. In general terms, the priorities for acute treatment must be safety, resolution of psychotic symptoms, and facilitation of long-term recovery.

Safety

In the context of treating patients with psychosis, safety must be ensured for the patients, their families, staff, and the community at large. Emergency administration of medications is just one component of the successful management of potentially dangerous patients. The provision of experienced nursing staff; a safe, closely monitored environment; and judicious use of seclusion and restraint are also very important.

Resolution of Psychotic Symptoms

Medications must be prescribed in a way that is effective at resolving the psychosis. The principal goal of antipsychotic medication is to resolve the symptoms of an acute psychotic episode: hallucinations, delusions, thought disorder, and disorganized behavior. From the outset, it is important that this goal be differentiated from that of behavioral control. Although the latter is also critical and frequently relevant to the management of acutely psychotic patients, the pharmacological approach to managing violent, agitated psychotic patients differs in important ways. This has been a source of confusion, in large part because antipsychotic medications have in the past served a dual purpose in controlling both psychosis and disturbed behavior. This has led to a lack of clarity in conceptualizing the optimal dose of antipsychotic medication required to treat patients with acute psychosis. If one uses the strategy of choosing an antipsychotic dose that will also reliably control agitation, one can expect that major problems (e.g., akathisia, parkinsonism, and dystonia) in tolerating medications will commonly occur. For this reason, it is best to separate out these two components of treatments. Agitation can usually be managed with benzodiazepines; antipsychotic medications are only needed in more extreme emergencies for the control of agitation itself. Antipsychotic medication can then be titrated with the sole purpose of controlling psychosis.

Facilitation of Long-Term Recovery

Treatment should be provided in a way that facilitates the engagement of the patient in his or her treatment and maximizes the patient's compliance with ongoing medication. It is absolutely critical that the short-term goals be met in a way that will not sacrifice the attainment of long-term recovery. It is not hard to imagine that the dual goals of achieving safety and resolving psychosis may be pursued with a degree of rapidity and aggressiveness that may jeopardize the patient's future treatment alliance. Initiating treatment in a way that facilitates long-term engagement may be a substantial challenge, particularly because a patient's first experience with treatment may well involve intramuscular injections, physical restraint, involuntary treatment, and acute dystonia and akathisia.

When Should Antipsychotic Medication Be Started?

The optimal timing for initiating antipsychotic medication should be given careful consideration. The first experience that a psychotic patient has with health professionals is of critical importance. If the encounter is well managed, it can lead to a dramatic transformation of the patient's mental health over the ensuing weeks. If the patient is not engaged satisfactorily with treatment, the next opportunity to treat may be months or even years away. It is not uncommon for patients to experience psychotic symptoms for a number of years before they finally find themselves in treatment. By this point, many patients have become socially isolated and marginal and have experienced much failure in attaining their developmentally appropriate social, educational, and vocational goals. Intervening as early as possible in the course of illness may well limit the disability the individual experiences. There is also accumulating evidence that the psychosis itself may be more difficult to treat if left untreated for an extended period of time (Loebel et al. 1992; Wyatt 1991). For this reason, it is extremely important that patients get quickly connected with a treatment team, either in the hospital or in the community.

Many patients experiencing a first episode of psychosis first present to an emergency department, where a determination should be made whether emergency intervention is required. Patients are sometimes sent home without follow-up examination because the acuteness of their presentation is not considered to be severe enough to warrant urgent treatment even though one of the goals of early treatment is to prevent patients from progressing to a stage of acuteness that requires emergency intervention. The opportunity to intervene early in the course of illness may be missed if the threshold for urgent admission into the treatment system is set too high.

Problems may arise because antipsychotic treatment is delayed but also because it is initiated too hastily. Patients who are cooperative and accepting of treatment are sometimes prescribed the same medication regimen that would usually be given to extremely agitated patients. There may be several reasons why this happens. Acute psychosis is frightening to all involved, and staff members may respond to even the most cooperative patients with a strong desire to eradicate all evidence of psychosis as rapidly as possible. Others may be used to prescribing antipsychotic medication in doses that will reliably control severe agitation. Such doses are associated with a high risk of akathisia and acute dystonia, side effects that are likely to be more frequent in these younger patients (Aguilar et al. 1994; Keepers and Casey 1991).

There are clearly situations in which antipsychotic medication should be prescribed within hours of presentation, but this should be the exception rather than the rule. An appropriate balance should be reached for each patient. Because the psychotic symptoms usually have been present for many months before presentation, there is usually time for the treatment team to review the treatment plan with the patient and family before initiating treatment with antipsychotic medication. It is not unreasonable to expect that if medical treatment is to be provided for a serious and potentially chronic medical condition, time must be spent establishing the diagnosis, educating the patient and his or her family, and reviewing the risks and benefits of medical treatment. Accepting the diagnosis of schizophrenia or schizophreniform disorder may take a great deal of time for both patients and families. However, one can usually get to the point at which antipsychotic medications can be prescribed within a few days of presentation. Benzodiazepines may be useful for patients with difficulties with sleep or mild agitation in the intervening period. In today's managed care environment, it may seem as though the top priority is to resolve the psychosis as quickly as possible so that the patient can be discharged in the minimum number of days. Although prompt resolution of the psychosis is an important priority, it is most critical that it be done in a way that maximizes the likelihood of engaging the patient sufficiently to ensure the type of long-term compliance necessary for managing a chronic illness.

It is becoming increasingly common to treat patients in their first episode of schizophrenia as outpatients. This may be feasible, particularly if there are supportive family members available to provide close supervision. The clinician should be confident that it is safe for the patient and the family for the patient to remain at home. When suicidal ideation or threatening behavior is evident, the hospital is a more appropriate setting for treatment. A hospital setting also affords the treatment team an opportunity to evaluate the clinical features of the illness and the patient's level of functioning. This may be particularly important if there is uncertainty about the diagnosis. It is safe to assume that to ensure compliance with treatment, patients need close monitoring, whether they are in a hospital or at home. Patients may agree to take medications on an outpatient basis but may be too ambivalent, disorganized, or paranoid to follow through. Titration of medication doses can also be quite complicated. It can be very traumatic for a newly treated patient to experience acute akathisia or dystonia while at home. Careful dose titration, liberal use of anticholinergic medication, and the prescription of atypical antipsychotic agents may facilitate successful treatment at home.

How Much Medication is Necessary?

Although antipsychotic medication is imperative in the treatment of a patient with a first episode of psychosis, there has been uncertainty about the amount of medication that is optimal. Ever since the introduction of antipsychotic medications in the 1950s, there has been considerable controversy over what constitutes an optimal dosage range for these agents. Much of the interest in the field has been in determining what constitutes an adequate trial of antipsychotic medication for those who are responding poorly—that is, the dosage at which one could say with confidence that there is no point increasing the dose any further. However, the more salient question in treating patients in their first episode is: What is the minimum effective dose for a given individual? Over the past decade, a consensus seemed to be emerging that dosages in the range of 10–20 mg of haloperidol per day (i.e., 500–1,000 chlorpromazine equivalents per day) would be sufficient for most patients with schizophrenia (Baldessarini et al. 1988; Bollini et al. 1994; Carpenter and Buchanan 1994). Dosages in this range were used in the first studies of treatment response in first-episode schizophrenia. The Scottish First Episode Schizophrenia Study (Scottish Schizophrenia Research Group 1987) involved treating patients with either pimozide, 10–40 mg/day (mean dose, 18.8 mg) or flupenthixol, 10–50 mg/day (mean dose, 20 mg). At the end of 5 weeks, 63% of patients were defined as responders; however, 78% of pimozide-treated patients and 85% of flupenthixol-treated patients required antiparkinsonian medications.

The landmark first episode study by Lieberman et al. (1993) incorporated similar dosages into their standard treatment algorithm, which involved starting all patients with a first episode of schizophrenia on 20 mg/day of fluphenazine hydrochloride (i.e., 1,000 chlorpromazine equivalents per day). Although treatment was associated with a remarkable 86% recovery rate in the first year, 62% of patients experienced extrapyramidal symptoms (EPS), including dystonia in 36%, akathisia in 18%, and parkinsonism in 24%. These studies require us to ask whether it is possible to achieve comparable response rates with doses of medication that would lead to lower rates of EPS.

The body of literature supporting dosing in this range was brought into question by the seminal study by McEvoy et al. (1991). This study was undertaken to investigate whether the "neuroleptic threshold" approach could be used to individualize the dosing of antipsychotic medication for the acute treatment of schizophrenia. A total of 106 patients were treated in this protocol, and 32 were being treated for the first time. In operationalizing this method, McEvoy et al. increased the dose of haloperidol every third day until the first signs of parkinsonian rigidity emerged. Whereas the mean "neuroleptic threshold dose" for those who had received previous treatment was 4.3 mg/day, those who were receiving treatment for the first time reached threshold at 2.1 mg/day. Dosages were then held at this level until the end of the first 24 days of the study. At this point, patients were randomized to either remain on their neuroleptic threshold dose or to be increased to a level 2–10 times their threshold dose (5–20 mg/day) for another 2 weeks. Increasing the dose in the second phase of the study did not lead to greater improvement than continuing at the "neuroleptic threshold" dose, irrespective of whether patients had responded well in the first phase of the study. This study challenged the prevailing dosing practices for antipsychotic medication and raised the question of whether patients being treated for the first time might require even smaller doses of medication.

After publication of the McEvoy study, our group (Zhang-Wong et al. 1999) became interested in determining the dosages of antipsychotic medication that would be optimal for the treatment of a patient having his or her first episode of psychosis. Patients were started on haloperidol at 2 mg/day for the first week. The dosage was increased incrementally on a weekly basis to 5, 10, and finally 20 mg/day until patients reached a dose at which they either had evidence of EPS or clinical improvement defined as improvement on the Positive and Negative Syndrome Scale for Schizophrenia (PANSS; Kay et al. 1987) total score of greater than 15%. Thirty-six patients were enrolled in the study; 15 were maintained at 2 mg/day (2 had EPS), 11 were maintained at 5 mg/day (6 had EPS), 7 were maintained at 10 mg/day (7 had EPS), and 3 were maintained at 20 mg/day (1 had EPS). By the end of the fourth week of the study, those who were maintained on 2 mg/day showed an average of 62% improvement on the PANSS compared with 47%, 27%, and 31% improvement for those treated with 5, 10, and 20 mg, respectively (Figure 4–1). Plasma haloperidol levels were also obtained. A total of 74% of those meeting criteria for response at 4 weeks had plasma haloperidol levels lower than 5 ng/mL, the usually quoted lower limit of the therapeutic range for haloperidol levels (Van Putten et al. 1990). Those maintained at a level of 2 mg/day had mean plasma haloperidol levels of 1.6±0.7 ng/mL.

Although interpretation of this study is necessarily constrained by its small sample size and its lack of a fixed-dose design, a number of important insights can be derived by carefully reviewing the data. Many patients have a substantial response to small doses of antipsychotic medication and are spared EPS; this is entirely consistent with the study by McEvoy et al. (1991). Although it is common in clinical practice to increase the dose of medication until a satisfactory response is achieved, this study demonstrates that by maintaining the dose at a level when early evidence of response has taken place, further response can be expected to occur with additional time. The greatest improvement was seen in those treated with the lowest doses of medication. Although it is possible that this is an artifact of study design (i.e., those who responded to the lowest dose stayed at their effective dose for the longest period of time), there are other possible explanations. Samples of patients in their first ep-

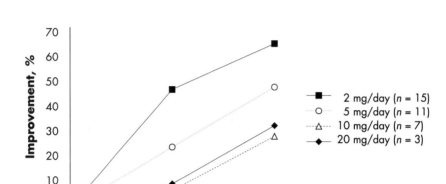

Figure 4–1. Percent improvement on total Positive and Negative Syndrome Scale for Schizophrenia score over 4 weeks for patients stabilized at each of the haloperidol dosage levels specified.
Source. Zhang-Wong et al. 1999. Used with permission.

isode should theoretically include those who are representative of the full spectrum of severity and responsiveness seen in schizophrenia. This is in contrast to the samples usually recruited for treatment studies in schizophrenia; less responsive patients are likely to be overrepresented in such studies. Many highly responsive patients have a full response to low doses of medication without having to reach the neuroleptic threshold. Some patients do not respond and end up receiving higher doses of medication. Such patients may be less responsive overall and have a less than complete resolution of symptoms despite receiving higher doses of medication. That patients who respond well to low doses of antipsychotic medication may represent a group with a less severe form of the illness is supported by our recent magnetic resonance imaging finding that patients who required larger doses of haloperidol had smaller volumes of cortical gray matter than those who were successfully treated with 2 mg/ day of haloperidol (Zipursky et al. 1998).

A fixed-dose design would have allowed us to address the question of whether the patients who ended up taking higher doses of haloperidol would have done just as well if they had been left at the lower doses. However, there are also problems in interpreting fixed-dose studies.

Fixed-dose studies allow one to identify the dose level at which the greatest average level of response is achieved. If some patients do require larger doses, then it is likely that larger doses will capture a greater percentage of responders than lower doses. This will result in a higher average degree of response in the higher-dose groups. This does not mean that those who would have responded to lower doses will show greater improvement when taking the higher ones (Freudenreich and McEvoy 1995).

We were very much struck by the low doses and low blood levels at which many patients in the study experienced substantial clinical response. It was initially unclear how this could be best understood. We therefore undertook a second study to determine the extent to which low doses of haloperidol (2 mg/day) result in occupancy of dopamine D_2 receptors in the brain. D_2 occupancy was measured with positron emission tomography (PET) by the binding of the radioligand (11 C)-raclopride to available D_2 receptors in the caudate nucleus and putamen (Kapur et al. 1996). Work by Nordstrom et al. (1993) has suggested that antipsychotic response is likely to take place if 70% or more of D_2 receptors are occupied, but EPS is likely to occur at occupancies of greater than 80%. We treated seven patients receiving treatment for a first episode of schizophrenia with haloperidol 2 mg/day and measured the resultant D_2 receptor occupancy and clinical response at 2 weeks. Patients had a mean D_2 receptor occupancy of 67% and mean improvement in positive and negative symptoms of 51% and 49%, respectively (Kapur et al. 1996). This study clearly established that 2 mg/day of haloperidol is likely to result in levels of D_2 receptor occupancy that fall within the range believed to be associated with clinical response.

The excellent response that many patients have to this dose of haloperidol gives rise to a number of critical questions. Will increasing the degree of D_2 receptor occupancy beyond this level enhance clinical response or only increase the likelihood of causing EPS? The results of the study by McEvoy et al. (1991) suggest that only the latter is likely to be true. Is it possible that response can be achieved at even lower levels of D_2 receptor occupancy? We recently addressed this question using a randomized, double-blind design that involved assigning patients receiving treatment for a first episode of psychosis to either 1.0 or 2.5 mg/day of haloperidol for a period of 2 weeks (Kapur et al. 2000b). Twenty-two patients underwent (11 C)-raclopride PET scanning to determine the degree of D_2 receptor occupancy achieved after 2 weeks of treatment. The patients who did not respond to treatment were then treated with haloperidol 5 mg/day for an additional 2 weeks. Patients were considered to be responders if they were rated on the Clinical Global Impressions–Improvement Scale (Guy 1976) as being "much improved" or "very much improved." The findings from this study are shown in Figure 4–2.

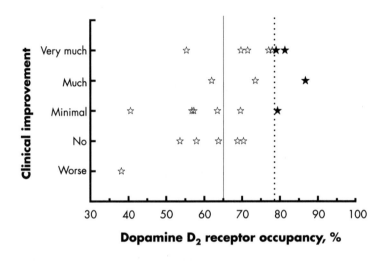

Figure 4–2. Improvement at 2 weeks for patients randomized to haloperidol 1.0 or 2.5 mg/day. The likelihood of responding was enhanced for those patients whose dopamine D_2 receptor occupancy was greater than 65% (*vertical solid line*). Extrapyramidal symptoms (EPS) were seen in those patients whose occupancy was greater than 78% (*vertical dotted line*). Patients who experienced EPS or akathisia are marked with *black stars*.
Source. Kapur et al. 2000b. Used with permission.

In this study, D_2 occupancies varied between 38% and 87%, with the mean occupancies for the 1- and 2.5-mg group being 59% and 75%, respectively. Seven of 9 patients treated with 2.5 mg/day responded to treatment compared with 3 of 13 treated with 1 mg/day. Although there does not appear to be a clear D_2 receptor occupancy threshold below which response cannot occur, it appeared from this study that the probability of responding was enhanced by having an occupancy level above 65%; 80% of initial responders were above this level in contrast to 67% of nonresponders who were below. Of the 12 nonresponders who had their dosage raised to 5 mg/day, 6 of 7 patients whose D_2 receptor occupancy had been below 65% responded, but only 1 of 4 who had initial occupancy over 65% responded. One nonresponder discontinued the study after having an acute dystonic reaction after his first 5-mg dose. Threshold levels were also determined for prolactin elevations and EPS. Although D_2 occupancies above 72% were associated with an 86% risk of prolactin elevation, those below this level had a 15% risk. Patients who experienced EPS or akathisia had significantly higher D_2 receptor occupancies than those without (79.7% vs. 63.8%; $P=0.04$); all patients who experienced EPS or akathisia had occupancies of greater than 78%.

Taken together, these data suggest that to maximize the likelihood of response while minimizing the likelihood of significant adverse effects, D_2 occupancy should be within the very narrow window of 65%–72%. Given the substantial interindividual variability in metabolism of haloperidol, it is not surprising that a large percentage of patients who improve with haloperidol experience significant adverse effects. Plasma haloperidol levels would be expected to provide a much better estimate of D_2 receptor occupancy than dose alone. In fact, we have found that plasma haloperidol levels explain 86% of the variance in D_2 receptor occupancy (Kapur et al. 1997). Plasma haloperidol levels can then be used to accurately predict D_2 receptor occupancy using the formula:

$$\% \ D_2 \text{ receptor occupancy} = 100 \times [\text{haloperidol}]/([\text{haloperidol}]+0.43)$$

where 0.43 is the concentration of haloperidol that results in 50% D_2 receptor occupancy (ED50) (Kapur et al. 1997). If the estimated D_2 receptor occupancy were within or above the 65%–72% range, one would expect further increases in dose to be more likely to result in side effects than in additional clinical benefit. Although this assertion should be fully tested in clinical trials, the studies by McEvoy et al. (1991) and Kapur et al. (1997) support this prediction. Whether the therapeutic window is larger for atypical agents remains an important question.

The observation that many patients experiencing a first episode of psychosis respond to low doses of antipsychotic medication (with moderate degrees of D_2 receptor occupancy) has important consequences for planning not only acute treatment but maintenance treatment as well. If patients respond to low doses with little or no side effects, there is no compelling reason to embark on a dose reduction strategy for maintenance treatment. Patients can easily be maintained on the dose to which they responded, thereby avoiding the trial-and-error approach to selecting an optimal maintenance dose. This is what is done in clinical practice in our program. A long-standing paradox in the treatment of patients with schizophrenia has been the observation that patients can be maintained on doses of long-acting depot medications that are associated with very low plasma levels even though acute treatment has involved using doses associated with much higher levels. A parsimonious explanation is that most patients also respond acutely to these low doses. It remains to be determined how often and for how long occupancies at this level need to be achieved to be effective for acute and maintenance treatment (Nyberg et al. 1995).

How clear is it that patients receiving treatment for a first episode of psychosis require lower doses of antipsychotic medication than patients with chronic schizophrenia? The study by McEvoy et al. (1991) suggested that first-episode patients required a mean dose of 2.1 mg/day compared with 3.4 mg/day for patients with multiple episodes. Stone et al. (1995) recently demonstrated that patients with relapses of chronic schizophrenia responded as well to 4 mg/day as to 10 or 40 mg/day. Similarly, Janicek et al. (1997) demonstrated that acutely relapsed patients randomized to receive haloperidol at plasma levels below the therapeutic range (mean dose, 3.3 mg/day) responded as well as patients treated within or above the therapeutic range (mean doses 25 and 51 mg/day, respectively). Although patients receiving treatment for a first episode of schizophrenia may be expected, on average, to be more responsive to low doses of medications, these studies suggest doses of haloperidol in the 2–5-mg range are also very effective for many patients with an established chronic course. In the face of poor response to this dose range, there is conflicting evidence about the value of increasing the dose beyond this range (Janicek et al. 1997; McEvoy 1991). The study by Kapur et al. (2000b) suggests that one can certainly expect a significant increase in side effects if this option is selected.

Should Atypical Antipsychotic Agents Be the First-Line Treatment?

If the premise is accepted that early intervention is key to optimizing the long-term outcome of patients with schizophrenia, then it is will be equally clear that it is important that the most effective medications be used at this stage of the illness. If a new medication will increase the extent of recovery, it hardly makes sense to limit use of such a medication to those with only the most severe and treatment-resistant forms of the illness. Evidence should be gathered to support the use of atypical antipsychotic medication in first-episode schizophrenia. What sort of evidence do we need? I believe that a strong argument should be made for the use of atypical antipsychotic medications as first-line agents for the treatment of first-episode schizophrenia if one or more of the following can be proven:

1. They are more effective at resolving the clinical features of schizophrenia (including positive symptoms, negative symptoms, disorganization, and cognitive deficits).
2. They lead to a superior outcome.

   Or, in the presence of equal but not better efficacy,

3. They are better tolerated.
4. They are associated with a greater degree of compliance.
5. They carry a reduced risk of tardive dyskinesia (TD).

Given these criteria, one could argue that clozapine should be the first-line treatment. That it carries little or no risk of TD (Meltzer 1992) is, in itself, a very compelling reason to seriously consider its use in this population. It also carries a very low risk of acute EPS. Clozapine is an effective antipsychotic medication that is superior for those who respond poorly to typical antipsychotic agents (Kane et al. 1988). Several factors, however, limit clozapine use in the first episode: 1) it has not been proven to be more efficacious in this patient group; given the high remission rate seen in this group with typical agents (Lieberman et al. 1993) it may be very difficult to establish the clinical superiority of clozapine; 2) the increased risk of agranulocytosis (Honigfeld et al. 1998) has to be weighed against the advantage vis à vis TD; 3) blood monitoring is burdensome and intrusive, particularly at this phase of the illness; and 4) clozapine is poorly tolerated by a substantial number of patients because of sedation, hypotension, drooling, and urinary incontinence. Clinical trials are currently under way to determine whether efficacy arguments support clozapine use as a first-line agent for patients with first-episode schizophrenia.

If it were possible to develop a drug with the advantages of clozapine without the risk of agranulocytosis or problems in tolerability, it would be a great stride forward. A new generation of atypical antipsychotic agents (i.e., risperidone, olanzapine, quetiapine, ziprasadone) has been introduced with this potential promise. At the outset, it should be asked whether the D_2 binding properties of these medications in vivo are more comparable with those observed with typical antipsychotic agents or with clozapine. We have demonstrated that both risperidone and olanzapine in their usual dosage ranges (i.e., 2–6 and 5–20 mg/day, respectively) lead to 60%–80% D_2 receptor occupancy (Kapur et al. 1995, 1998) (Figure 4–3). These levels are comparable with those observed with low-dose typical antipsychotic agents (Kapur et al. 1996, 1997, 2000b) and higher than those seen with clozapine (Kapur et al. 1999). At the same time, it is certainly clear that both olanzapine and risperidone possess potent 5-HT_2–blocking activity, much like clozapine (Kapur et al. 1999). Given the high degree of D_2 blockade seen with each of these agents, the question of whether these agents have substantial advantages in terms of acute EPS and TD needs to be carefully examined.

We have recently demonstrated that clinical doses of quetiapine result in very low levels of D_2 receptor occupancy (0%–27%) as assessed 12 hours postdose (Kapur et al. 2000a). When D_2 receptor occupancy was measured 2–3 hours postdose, quetiapine was observed to be blocking many more receptors (58%–64%). Quetiapine's short half-life and very low affinity for the D_2 receptor underlie this transient D_2 binding. Quetiapine, however, appears to have efficacy as an antipsychotic agent despite this very transient occupancy of D_2 receptors. Clozapine also binds very transiently at the D_2 receptor, a feature that may contribute to its atypicality. This may explain why both clozapine and quetiapine are associated with very low risks of EPS and may, in part, explain clozapine's superior efficacy. If persistent high levels of D_2 blockade are not necessary for antipsychotic response, it is conceivable that there may be a significant clinical advantage to treating patients with those medications whose D_2 occupancy is more transient. Further studies are needed to evaluate this possibility.

Does other evidence support the use of atypical antipsychotic agents for first-episode schizophrenia? At this point, it should be clarified that the critical question is not whether these new medications are effective in the first episode but whether the advantages that they offer are great enough to outweigh their disadvantages (e.g., weight gain and cost). It is for this reason that the American Psychiatric Association's (1997) guidelines for treating schizophrenia include atypical agents (other than clozapine) as potential agents to be used in the first line of treatment. Should these agents, however, become the treatment of choice for first-episode schizophrenia, with older typical agents relegated to a secondary role for poor responders? What is the evidence to support this view?

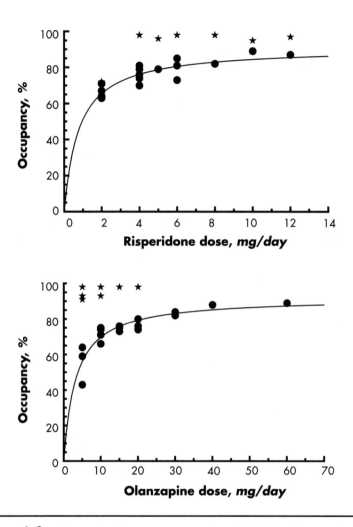

Figure 4–3. Dopamine D_2 receptor occupancy (*circles*) and serotonin 5-HT$_2$ receptor occupancy (*stars*) as a function of dose for risperidone (*top*) and olanzapine (*bottom*).

Source. Kapur et al. 1999. Used with permission.

Efficacy

This question has been examined in a number of trials involving risperidone. Kopala et al. (1996) treated 22 patients with a first episode of schizophrenia with risperidone in an open study and found it to be effective and well tolerated. Keshavan et al. (1998) treated 16 first-episode patients with risperidone and compared their responses with those of first-episode patients from their center who had been involved in an earlier study of low-dose haloperidol treatment. Symptom improvement over 4 weeks was comparable between the two groups. The risperidone group was significantly less likely to receive anticholinergic medications, but no difference was observed in the severity of EPS. In a large multinational, multicenter, randomized, double-blind trial, Emsley (1999) studied 183 patients (171 with schizophreniform disorder and 12 with schizophrenia) who were treated with either risperidone or haloperidol for 6 weeks. Dosages of these medications were titrated between 2 and 16 mg/day over the course of the study. At the end of the study, the mean dose of risperidone used was 6.1 mg/day compared with 5.6 mg/day of haloperidol. Improvement in positive and negative symptoms was comparable for the two groups. The incidence of EPS was high in both groups: 54% for risperidone and 83% for haloperidol. Risperidone caused significantly less EPS than haloperidol and was associated with less frequent use of anticholinergic medication and a lower dropout rate. It may be questioned whether any meaningful differences would have been eliminated if somewhat lower doses of each of the medications had been used or if prophylactic anticholinergic medication had been prescribed.

Although no specific first-episode studies have been reported that involve olanzapine, an analysis (Sanger et al. 1999) has been published of all patients receiving treatment for a first episode of schizophrenia, schizoaffective disorder, or schizophreniform disorder who had been involved in a large, prospective, multicenter, double-blind study comparing olanzapine with haloperidol. Eighty-three patients meeting criteria were studied, of whom 59 had received treatment with olanzapine and 24 with haloperidol. Mean modal doses for olanzapine and haloperidol were 11.6 and 10.8 mg, respectively. In terms of medication response, 67.2% of olanzapine-treated patients had improvement of 40% or more as measured by the Brief Psychiatric Rating Scale (BPRS) compared with 29.2% of haloperidol-treated patients. Patients treated with olanzapine had greater reduction on their BPRS total and negative (but not positive) score as well as on the PANSS total and PANSS positive (but not PANSS negative) score. Of those receiving olanzapine, 72.9% completed the study compared with 37.5% of those who received haloperidol. Patients receiving haloperidol were more likely to discontinue the study because of an adverse event (15.7%) than those who received olanzapine (1.7%). Haloperidol treatment was associated with significantly greater akathisia, EPS, and prolactin elevation. Treatment with olanzapine, on the other hand, was associated with an average weight gain of 4.1 kg over the 6-week period compared with 0.5 kg for those treated with haloperidol. At a first glance, it is certainly tempting to interpret this data as compelling evidence that olanzapine does, in fact, have clear advantages over haloperidol for the treatment of first-episode psychosis in terms of response rate, degree of symptom improvement, incidence of EPS, and treatment compliance. As in the case of the risperidone studies quoted previously, it is difficult to know whether these advantages would remain significant if more appropriate comparison doses of haloperidol had been used.

Outcome

There is no evidence to date that treatment with any of the new atypical agents results in substantial advantages in longer-term outcome. Trials addressing this question are currently under way.

Tolerability

Studies involving patients with chronic schizophrenia have demonstrated that both risperidone (Chouinard et al. 1993; Marder and Meibach 1994) and olanzapine (Beasley Jr. et al. 1996; Tollefson et al. 1997b) are associated with less EPS than haloperidol. However, the reference doses of haloperidol used are well beyond the low dose range now used in first-episode schizophrenia and are not comparable in terms of D_2 receptor occupancy with the doses of the atypical agents used (Kapur et al. 1999). It may well be that even with proper comparison doses of haloperidol, an advantage may still be present for the new agents. However, if the risk of EPS becomes very small with low-dose haloperidol, then the importance of this advantage will continue to be debatable. Quetiapine and olanzapine also possess significant advantages in terms of their relatively reduced risk of causing prolactin elevation (Beasley Jr. et al. 1996; Kleinberg et al. 1999) and the amenorrhea, galactorrhea, gynecomastia, and sexual dysfunction that may follow from it. Whatever advantages the new atypical antipsychotic agents have in terms of a reduced risk of EPS and prolactin elevation must be balanced against the increased likelihood of other side effects, particularly weight gain (Allison et al. 1999; Wirshing et al. 1999), which is associated with its own substantial social and health costs.

Compliance

One would expect that long-term compliance would be greater with the new atypical medications if they lead to fewer side effects. This remains to be established. In our experience, many patients receiving low-dose typical agents can be successfully treated with minimal side effects. Nonetheless, patients frequently become noncompliant for reasons other than medication side effects. Although eliminating medication side effects is critical in treating all patients, including those with first-episode schizophrenia, it is important to understand that eliminating one common cause of noncompliance does not prevent other substantial causes from becoming clinically relevant. Accepting that one has a chronic mental illness and that one requires ongoing medical treatment are formidable tasks for patients in their first episode, even in the absence of side effects from medication.

Tardive Dyskinesia

If any new antipsychotic medication can be demonstrated to be as effective as typical agents but associated with a substantially reduced incidence of TD, it will clearly represent a breakthrough in the management of patients with schizophrenia. As TD develops over the course of many months and years, such differences need to be investigated with longer-term prospective studies of first-episode patients. Evidence from short-term acute treatment studies of risperidone (Marder and Meibach 1994), olanzapine (Tollefson et al. 1997b), and quetiapine (Small et al. 1997) have, in general, found little difference in the severity of TD compared with haloperidol. Chouinard (1995) has suggested, on the basis of an analysis of the Canadian Multicentre Risperidone Study, that risperidone at a dosage of 6 mg/day may have a beneficial effect on TD in comparison with both placebo and haloperidol (20 mg/day). Similarly, Tollefson et al. (1997a) reported that patients who had been involved in treatment studies of olanzapine versus haloperidol for a median of 237 and 203 days, respectively, were less likely to develop treatment-emergent TD if they had been assigned to the olanzapine group. TD was present in 1.0% of olanzapine patients in the final two Abnormal Involuntary Movement Scale (AIMS) assessments, compared with 4.6% of haloperidol-treated patients. Again, interpretation of this data is limited by the substantially higher comparison doses of haloperidol (mean dose, 14.7 mg/day) than olanzapine (mean dose, 14.4 mg/day). Finally, Tran et al. (1997) compared the incidence of treatment-emergent TD in a 28-week study of 339 patients randomized to olanzapine (modal dose, 17.2 mg/day) or risperidone (modal dose, 7.2 mg/day). Patients receiving risperidone were more likely to have developed TD as assessed at the last visit than patients receiving olanzapine (10.7% vs. 4.6%, respectively). The interpretation of this finding is also limited by the somewhat higher relative doses of risperidone prescribed. Although it is generally believed that duration of exposure to antipsychotic medication is a much more important risk factor for the development of TD than dosage, the evidence supporting this view is largely based on data from a period when relative large doses of antipsychotic medication were standard. It is conceivable that within the higher dosage range, there is no effect of dose on the risk of TD but that such an effect would be detectable if patients being treated in the lower dosage range were included.

It is not yet possible to conclude that any of the atypical agents is superior to haloperidol for patients experiencing a first episode of psychosis in terms of either efficacy or outcome. Prospective longitudinal treatment studies of first-episode patients that include appropriate comparison doses of typical antipsychotic agents are needed to resolve these questions. Such studies are currently under way and should be able to clarify the potential benefits of the atypical agents with regard to compliance and TD. It does seem highly likely that one or more of the atypical agents will prove to be associated with less akathisia and less acute EPS than are observed with low doses of typical antipsychotic agents. If the risk of such events is relatively small with low doses of typical agents, this consideration will need to be weighed against the increased likelihood of other adverse events with the atypical antipsychotic agents, particularly weight gain. Finally, it should be kept in mind that haloperidol may not be the optimal drug to be compared with the new atypicals; if a mid-potency typical antipsychotic agent (e.g., perphenazine, loxapine) were chosen as the comparison drug, it might be more difficult to demonstrate that atypical agents are associated with less EPS (Hoyberg et al. 1993).

What If the Patient Does Not Respond to Treatment?

Although most first-episode patients respond very well to treatment, there are many who respond poorly or incompletely. Poor response represents an important opportunity for the treatment team to review the diagnosis, the patient's level of compliance with the medication regimen, and the adequacy of the trial (i.e., dose and duration). There is considerable variability in the time to response that is seen in first-episode patients: although some respond robustly in days, others may take many months. If substantial response is observed to be taking place over the first month of treatment, it may well be that further improvement will require additional time rather than a change in medication or dose. With the current trend for relatively low doses in first-episode patients, there will undoubtedly be some patients who fail to respond because they have been treated with inadequate doses; dose increases may then be important. As a general rule, there is little value in increasing the dose to the point at which the patient experiences akathisia or EPS. With the range of typical and atypical antipsychotic agents available today, there is no need for these side effects to be tolerated on an ongoing basis. In our program, a new trial of medication would be recommended if patients have not experienced significant improvement after a 4–6-week trial at an optimal dose of medication. If a determination is made that a patient has responded poorly to a given trial of medication, a decision needs to be made about the next antipsychotic agent to be used. There is little research available to help in this decision. It is not known whether such patients should have multiple trials of different atypical or typical antipsychotic medications before clozapine is considered. In our experience, many patients respond well to the second trial; it cannot be determined whether this is best explained by differences in efficacy, side effects, or the effect of additional time.

The role of clozapine in managing first-episode patients who have responded poorly or incompletely remains to be fully clarified. Clozapine has been demonstrated to be superior for patients with treatment-resistant forms of illness (Kane et al. 1988). Szymanski et al. (1994) studied 10 first-episode patients who had responded poorly to sequential trials of three "typical" antipsychotic agents of three different biochemical classes. Their response to clozapine was comparable with that observed in the Kane et al. study: 3 of 10 patients met criteria for response. In treating first-episode patients, clozapine's major role does not seem to be in treating patients who are nonresponders. Rather, its role may well be in treating those who have improved with other medications but have been left with significant persisting psychotic symptoms. In our experience at the University of Toronto, many first-episode patients who would be considered partial responders to first- and second-line treatments have a very substantial degree of additional improvement when switched to clozapine. After poorly responding patients are given thorough trials of two or three different antipsychotic medications, clozapine should be considered. In such patients, clozapine can usually be initiated in the first 6–12 months of treatment. If clozapine is able to bring about a greater degree of response, it is important for the individual patient that this improvement be experienced sooner rather than later.

How Long Should the Patient Take Medication?

When a first episode of psychosis is successfully brought into remission, it is unavoidable that the clinician will be faced with the question of how long the patient needs to take medication. With the advent of low-dose treatment strategies, there is no longer much of a middle-road option of simply reducing the dose. A decision needs to be made on this issue; if the psychiatrist avoids dealing with the issue, it may be expected that the patient will ultimately make the decision. Current guidelines published by the American Psychiatric Association (1997) suggest that "a patient who has had only one episode of positive symptoms and has had no symptoms during the follow-up year of maintenance therapy may be considered for a trial period without medication" (p. 41). To determine whether it is advisable for an individual patient to discontinue medications, it is important to be aware of the literature's bearing on this critical issue.

Several studies have investigated the risk of relapse after a first episode of schizophrenia (for review, see Ram et al. 1992). It is important to distinguish between studies that include only remitted patients and those that include all patients. One would not usually consider discontinuing the medications of a first-episode patient who had a significant but incomplete antipsychotic response. The question of greatest salience is how medications affect the likelihood that a remitted patient will relapse.

Kane et al. (1982) studied the rate of relapse in 28 remitted patients who had had a first episode of schizophrenia. Patients were randomly assigned to treatment with fluphenazine or placebo and followed up for 1 year. Seven of 17 patients who received placebo relapsed within the year compared with none of the 11 who received fluphenazine. Rabiner et al. (1986) carried out a 1-year naturalistic follow-up study of 64 patients who had been hospitalized for their first psychotic episode. Of the 28 patients with schizophrenia, 8 had relapsed within the year; 18 patients with schizophrenia had stopped taking medications, including all 8 who had relapsed. Relapse rates increase as the duration of the follow-up period is increased. The 5-year follow-up of the Scottish First Episode Schizophrenia Study (Scottish Schizophrenia Research Group 1992) reported a relapse rate of 74%. Most recently, Robinson et al. (1999) reported on the 5-year follow-up of 104 first-episode patients studied at Hillside Hospital (Lieberman et al. 1992). By the end of the first year of follow-up, 16% had relapsed; the percentage increased to 54% at 2 years, 63% at 3 years, 75% at 4 years, and 82% at 5 years. Patients who were not taking antipsychotic medications were five times more likely to relapse than those who were taking medications.

Many remitted patients are keen to discontinue medication and express their commitment to resume medication if any signs of illness return. Perhaps patients could be trained to identify the early signs of relapse and restart medications in time to avoid the next psychotic episode. Although this certainly sounds compelling, the efficacy and safety of this approach should be demonstrated. There has been much interest in evaluating this type of targeted or intermittent treatment in multiepisode patients. The results of several randomized controlled trials have demonstrated that the rates of relapse and rehospitalization are substantially higher in patients receiving targeted treatment (Carpenter et al. 1990; Jolley et al. 1990). Whether this holds true for first-episode patients is not known. Given the evidence from studies of multiepisode patients, there is certainly reason for caution; nonetheless, because many patients will undoubtedly choose this option, there will be ample opportunity to evaluate its efficacy.

Taken together, the studies suggest that there is a 70%–90% risk of having a relapse after a first episode of schizophrenia and that patients who discontinue antipsychotic medications are at dramatically increased risk relative to those who continue on the medication. Although it can be argued that 10%–30% of patients may stay well without antipsychotic medication, it is important to keep in mind the enormous toll exacted with each relapse: results include the suffering involved in weeks or months of being psychotic, the destruction of relationships, job loss, school failure, social alienation, and financial problems. Recovery from a second episode may take longer than the initial recovery, and the degree of recovery may not be as robust (Lieberman 1996; Wiersma et al. 1998). How one factors this into an individual's decision to discontinue medications is challenging, to say the least. At this point, it is less than clear that discontinuing medications is justifiable from a risk–benefit perspective, particularly if medication side effects become an insignificant issue. Further work needs to address this important question directly.

Conclusions

Patients experiencing a first episode of schizophrenia must be treated as early as possible in their illness with the medications that are most effective and least likely to result in adverse effects. It is now clear that many patients can be treated successfully and comfortably with low doses of either typical agents or new atypical agents. We are well on our way to eliminating akathisia, parkinsonism, and dystonia as major problems in the treatment of patients with schizophrenia. In all likelihood, the advent of clozapine and newer atypical agents will greatly reduce—if not eliminate—the risk of TD. The greatest challenge that lies ahead is to determine which treatments offer the greatest benefit across the range of symptom, cognitive, and functional domains so that patients are afforded the best opportunity for a full recovery.

References

Aguilar EJ, Keshavan MS, Martinez-Quiles MD, et al: Predictors of acute dystonia in first-episode psychotic patients. Am J Psychiatry 151:1819–1821, 1994

Allison DB, Fontaine KR, Heo M, et al: The distribution of body mass index among individuals with and without schizophrenia. J Clin Psychiatry 60:215–220, 1999

American Psychiatric Association: Practice guideline for the treatment of patients with schizophrenia. Am J Psychiatry 154(suppl):1–63, 1997

Baldessarini R, Cohen B, Teicher M: Significance of neuroleptic dose and plasma level in the pharmacological treatment of psychoses. Arch Gen Psychiatry 45:79–91, 1988

Beasley Jr CM, Tollefson G, Tran P, et al: Olanzapine versus placebo and haloperidol: acute phase results of the North American double-blind olanzapine trial. Neuropsychopharmacology 14:111–123, 1996

Bollini P, Pampallona S, Orza MJ, et al: Antipsychotic drugs: is more worse? A meta-analysis of the published randomized control trials. Psychol Med 24:307–316, 1994

Carpenter WT, Buchanan RW: Schizophrenia. N Engl J Med 330:681–690, 1994

Carpenter WTJ, Hanlon TE, Heinrichs DW, et al: Continuous versus targeted medication in schizophrenic outpatients: outcome results. Am J Psychiatry 147:1138–1148, 1990

Chouinard G: Effects of risperidone in tardive dyskinesia: an analysis of the Canadian Multicentre Risperidone Study. J Clin Psychopharmacol 15(suppl):36–44, 1995

Chouinard G, Jones B, Remington G, et al: A Canadian multicenter placebo-controlled study of risperidone and haloperidol in the treatment of chronic schizophrenic patients. J Clin Psychopharmacol 13:25–40, 1993

Emsley RA: Risperidone in the treatment of first-episode psychotic patients: a double-blind multicenter study. Risperidone Working Group. Schizophr Bull 25:721–729, 1999

Freudenreich O, McEvoy JP: Added amantadine may diminish tardive dyskinesia in patients requiring continued neuroleptics (letter to the editor). J Clin Psychiatry 56:173, 1995

Guy W: Clinical Global Impression Scale, in ECDEU Assessment Manual for Psychopharmacology. Washington, DC, U.S. Public Health Service, 1976, pp 218–222

Honigfeld G, Arellano F, Sethi J, et al: Reducing clozapine-related morbidity and mortality: 5 years of experience with the Clozaril National Registry. J Clin Psychiatry 59:3–7, 1998

Hoyberg OJ, Fensbo C, Remvig J, et al: Risperidone versus perphenazine in the treatment of chronic schizophrenic patients with acute exacerbations. Acta Psychiatr Scand 88:395–402, 1993

Janicek PG, Javaid JI, Sharma RP, et al: A two-phase, double-blind randomized study of three haloperidol plasma levels for acute psychosis with reassignment of initial non-responders. Acta Psychiatr Scand 95:343–350, 1997

Jolley AG, Hirsch SR, Morrison E, et al: Trial of brief intermittent neuroleptic prophylaxis for selected schizophrenic outpatients: clinical and social outcomes at two years. BMJ 301:837–842, 1990

Kane JM, Rifkin A, Quitkin F, et al: Fluphenazine vs placebo in patients with remitted, acute first-episode schizophrenia. Arch Gen Psychiatry 39:70–73, 1982

Kane J, Honigfeld G, Singer J, et al: Clozapine for the treatment-resistant schizophrenic: a double-blind comparison with chlorpromazine. Arch Gen Psychiatry 45:789–796, 1988

Kapur S, Remington G, Zipursky RB, et al: The D2-dopamine receptor occupancy of risperidone and its relationship to extrapyramidal symptoms: a PET study. Life Sci 57:PL103–PL107, 1995

Kapur S, Remington G, Jones C, et al: High levels of dopamine D2 receptor occupancy with low dose haloperidol treatment: a PET study. Am J Psychiatry 153:948–950, 1996

Kapur S, Zipursky RB, Roy P, et al: The relationship between D2 receptor occupancy and plasma levels on low dose oral haloperidol: a PET study. Psychopharmacol (Berl) 131:148–152, 1997

Kapur S, Zipursky RB, Remington G, et al: 5-HT2 and D2 receptor occupancy of olanzapine in schizophrenia: a PET investigation. Am J Psychiatry 155:921–928, 1998

Kapur S, Zipursky RB, Remington G: Clinical and therapeutic implications of 5-HT2 and D2 receptor occupancy of clozapine, risperidone and olanzapine in schizophrenia. Am J Psychiatry 156:286–293, 1999

Kapur S, Zipursky R, Jones C, et al: A positron emission tomography study of quetiapine in schizophrenia: a preliminary finding of an antipsychotic effect with only transiently high dopamine D2 receptor occupancy. Arch Gen Psychiatry 57:553–559, 2000a

Kapur S, Zipursky R, Jones C, et al: The relationship between dopamine D(2) occupancy, clinical response, and side effects: a double-blind PET study of first episode schizophrenia. Am J Psychiatry 157:514–520, 2000b

Kay SR, Fiszbein A, Opler LA: The Positive and Negative Syndrome Scale (PANSS) for Schizophrenia. Schizophr Bull 13:261, 1987

Keepers GA, Casey DE: Use of neuroleptic-induced extrapyramidal symptoms to predict future vulnerability to side effects. Am J Psychiatry 148:85–89, 1991

Keshavan MS, Schooler NR, Sweeney JA, et al: Research and treatment strategies in first-episode psychoses. The Pittsburgh experience. Br J Psychiatry 172(suppl):60–65, 1998

Kleinberg DL, Davis JM, de Coster R, et al: Prolactin levels and adverse events in patients treated with risperidone. J Clin Psychopharmacol 19:57–61, 1999

Kopala LC, Fredrikson D, Good KP, et al: Symptoms in neuroleptic-naive, first-episode schizophrenia: response to risperidone. Biol Psychiatry 39:296–298, 1996

Lieberman JA: Pharmacotherapy for patients with first-episode, acute and refractory schizophrenia. Psychiatr Ann 26:515–518, 1996

Lieberman JA, Alvir J, Woerner M, et al: Prospective study of psychobiology in first-episode schizophrenia at Hillside Hospital. Schizophr Bull 18:351–371, 1992

Lieberman JA, Jody D, Geisler S, et al: Time course and biological correlates of treatment response in first-episode schizophrenia. Arch Gen Psychiatry 50:369–376, 1993

Loebel AD, Lieberman JA, Alvir JMJ, et al: Duration of psychosis and outcome in first episode schizophrenia. Am J Psychiatry 149:1183–1188, 1992

Marder SR, Meibach RC: Risperidone in the treatment of schizophrenia. Am J Psychiatry 151:825–835, 1994

McEvoy JP, Hogarty GE, Steingard S: Optimal dose of neuroleptic in acute schizophrenia: a controlled study of neuroleptic threshold and higher haloperidol dose. Arch Gen Psychiatry 48:739–745, 1991

Meltzer HY: Treatment of the neuroleptic-nonresponsive schizophrenic patient. Schizophr Bull 18:515–42, 1992

Nordstrom A-L, Farde L, Wiesel FA, et al: Central D2-dopamine receptor occupancy in relation to antipsychotic drug effect: a double-blind PET study of schizophrenic patients. Biol Psychiatry 33:237–235, 1993

Nyberg S, Farde L, Halldin C, et al: D2 dopamine receptor occupancy during low-dose treatment with haloperidol decanoate. Am J Psychiatry 152:173–178, 1995

Rabiner CJ, Wegner JT, Kane JM: Outcome study of first-episode psychosis, I: relapse rates after 1 year. Am J Psychiatry 143:1155–1158, 1986

Ram R, Bromet EJ, Eaton WW, et al: The natural course of schizophrenia: a review of first-admission studies. Schizophr Bull 18:185–207, 1992

Robinson D, Woerner MG, Alvir JM, et al: Predictors of relapse following response from a first episode of schizophrenia or schizoaffective disorder. Arch Gen Psychiatry 56:241–7, 1999

Sanger TM, Lieberman JA, Tohen M, et al: Olanzapine versus haloperidol treatment in first-episode psychosis. Am J Psychiatry 156:79–87, 1999

Scottish Schizophrenia Research Group: The Scottish first episode schizophrenia study, II. Treatment: pimozide versus flupenthixol. Br J Psychiatry 150:334–8, 1987

Scottish Schizophrenia Research Group: The Scottish first episode schizophrenia study, VIII. Five-year follow-up: clinical and psychosocial findings. Br J Psychiatry 161:496–500, 1992

Small JG, Hirsch SR, Arvanitis LA, et al: Quetiapine in patients with schizophrenia: a high- and low-dose double-blind comparison with placebo. Arch Gen Psychiatry 54:549–557, 1997

Stone CK, Garver DL, Griffith J, et al: Further evidence of a dose response threshold for haloperidol in psychosis. Am J Psychiatry 152:1210–1212, 1995

Szymanski S, Masiar S, Mayerhoff D, et al: Clozapine response in treatment-refractory first-episode schizophrenia. Biol Psychiatry 35:278–280, 1994

Tollefson GD, Beasley CM, Tamura RN, et al: Blind, controlled, long-term study of the comparative incidence of treatment-emergent tardive dyskinesia with olanzapine and haloperidol. Am J Psychiatry 154:1248–1254, 1997a

Tollefson GD, Beasley CM, Tran PV, et al: Olanzapine versus haloperidol in the treatment of schizophrenia and schizoaffective and schizophreniform disorders: results of an international collaborative trial. Am J Psychiatry 154:457–465, 1997b

Tran PV, Hamilton SH, Kuntz AJ, et al: Double-blind comparison of olanzapine versus risperidone in the treatment of schizophrenia and other psychotic disorders. J Clin Psychopharmacol 17:407–418, 1997

Van Putten T, Marder SR, Mintz J: A controlled dose comparison of haloperidol in newly admitted schizophrenic patients. Arch Gen Psychiatry 47:754–758, 1990

Wiersma D, Nienhuis FJ, Sloof CJ, Giel R: Natural course of schizophrenic disorders: a 15-year follow-up of a Dutch incidence cohort. Schizophr Bull 24:75–85, 1998

Wirshing DA, Wirshing WC, Kysar L, et al: Novel antipsychotics: comparison of weight gain liabilities. J Clin Psychiatry 60:358–63, 1999

Wyatt RJ: Neuroleptics and the natural course of schizophrenia. Schizophr Bull 17:325–351, 1991

Zhang-Wong J, Zipursky RB, Beiser M, et al: Optimal haloperidol dosage in first-episode psychosis. Can J Psychiatry 44:164–7, 1999

Zipursky RB, Zhang-Wong J, Lambe EK, et al: MRI correlates of treatment response in first episode psychosis. Schizophr Res 30:81–90, 1998

5

Meeting the Patient's Emotional Needs

Elizabeth McCay, R.N., Ph.D.

Kathryn Ryan, R.N., M.Sc.(N.)

Individuals recovering from a first episode of schizophrenia experience a spectrum of emotional responses that ranges from anxiety, depression, and low self-esteem to the devastating response of suicidality. Clearly, the onset of schizophrenia and its emotional sequelae have the capacity to significantly interfere with the young person's developmental trajectory, sense of self, and overall well being. Young people encountering a first episode of schizophrenia realize that they have a highly stigmatizing illness, which raises questions about their sense of competence, self-esteem, and future aspirations. Coping with the ongoing shame, stigma, and social withdrawal associated with mental illness presents one of the most arduous challenges to recovery. Concomitantly, young people with this illness are also vulnerable to the phenomenon of illness engulfment, which results in the self-concept's becoming increasingly organized around the illness and around the patient role. Ultimately, a redefinition of self is required for individuals recovering from first-episode schizo-

The group intervention research referred to in this chapter was supported by grants from the Ontario Mental Health Foundation and the Centre for Addiction and Mental Health.

phrenia, one that incorporates and accommodates the illness in a positive and realistic light yet resists the precarious risk of engulfment. Intervention strategies designed to minimize the secondary trauma and engulfment arising from the illness may prevent the insidious development of chronicity in this young, vulnerable population. This chapter reviews the spectrum of emotional responses experienced by individuals in the early phase of illness recovery, discusses the impact of stigma and its effects on self-concept, and provides an overview of relevant interventions and related outcomes.

Emotional Responses to Illness

> Like I had always looked down on mental institutions, like when I was in high school there was a guy who was 3 years ahead of me and he wound up in a hospital. And I would always look down on him, for just being in here, in a place like this. Then when I got here, it was like my life had ended. (Lally 1989, p. 259)

Young people experiencing a first episode of psychosis and first admission to a psychiatric hospital often feel completely devastated and overwhelmed. The symptoms of psychosis (e.g., persecutory delusions and auditory hallucinations) can evoke intense fear, anxiety, and loss of control. These reactions may be intensified because of the fact that treatment usually occurs in a psychiatric hospital and frequently involves involuntary hospitalization and, in some cases, forced sedation and restraint.

These aspects of the illness and treatment experience are potentially traumatizing to the young person and may compound feelings of helplessness and powerlessness. Indeed, some psychological responses experienced by these individuals are similar to psychological reactions experienced by trauma victims and include depression, reexperiencing traumatic aspects of the illness, negative self-attributes, emotional numbing and denial, and reduced resilience to stress (McGorry et al. 1991). It has also been suggested that the negative syndrome, characterized by a lack of motivation, apathy, and social withdrawal, may also be the result of a traumatic reaction to the experience of illness (McGorry et al. 1991; Plasky 1991).

The experience of hospitalization and first-episode psychosis raises questions for individuals about who they are, challenges their sense of competence and self-esteem, and leaves them feeling vulnerable and faced with an uncertain future. Whereas many patients may worry about becoming ill again and struggle with the unpredictable nature of the illness course, others may be firmly convinced they will never experience another episode and may stop treatment prematurely. Denial is a common emotional response that may reflect the individual's attempt to preserve self-esteem and a sense of competence and to resist the threat of self-stigmatization (Lally 1989; McGorry 1995). As individuals come to terms with illness, they often experience a sense of shock and disbelief as well as profound shame and alienation about having a highly stigmatizing illness. One young man described the impact of coming to terms with his illness thus:

> It wasn't until a month or so after being discharged from hospital that I began to see that it was very possible that something was biologically malfunctioning. And it was very difficult to accept because it meant accepting that somehow one was not well; one was not normal....It became another blow to my self-confidence.

Illness labels such as "schizophrenia" are frequently associated with a profound loss of hope for the future and an overwhelming sense of shame. We are currently carrying out a study to evaluate a group intervention designed to reduce engulfment and to promote the psychological and social adjustment of individuals recovering from a first episode of psychosis. In a test of the group intervention, individuals explored the meaning of their illness and expressed tremendous fear that labeling the illness or receiving a diagnosis such as schizophrenia would result in feeling stigmatized, misunderstood, and rejected. Participants preferred to refer to their illness as a nervous breakdown because of the stereotypes and stigma associated with the labels "schizophrenia" and "psychosis" (McCay et al. 1996). This is illustrated in the following quote:

> There's a huge stigma, either psychosis or schizophrenia. Both of these have serial killer kinds of origins and usually it's not a very congenial kind of thing, so "nervous breakdown" tends to show a person who is a bit sensitive or somehow sensitive to certain things and doesn't really mean they're scary...It shifts the perception from someone you should be afraid of to someone who isn't a threat.

In addition, one young man said he told a friend he had schizophrenia and then felt extremely anxious, as though he was experiencing a dissociative reaction. Through our discussion, it become clear that his reaction was a result of his profound fear he would be viewed as "less of a person" and "not on the same level" as others who are not ill.

It is not surprising that individuals often feel extremely sad and demoralized as they struggle to come to terms with their illness. These young adults, who typically have high hopes and expectations for themselves, are suddenly faced with the realization that they suffer from an illness that may interfere with their ability to achieve future aspirations. They may experience profound feelings of hopelessness and failure. Depression has been described as a major problem for individuals experiencing a first episode of schizophrenia, particularly during the initial acute phase and during the first year of illness (Addington et al. 1998; McGlashen and Carpenter 1976). Koreen et al. (1993) suggested that depression in first-episode schizophrenia may represent a core aspect of the acute illness or may occur as a subjective reaction to the experience of psychotic decompensation. The reported frequency of depression ranges from 22% to 80% (Addington et al. 1998). A recent study (Addington et al. 1998) suggested that individuals recovering from a first episode of schizophrenia are at greater risk of depression than individuals who have had multiple episodes of illness. Depression in individuals with schizophrenia has been cited as a risk factor for suicide (Drake and Sederer 1986). Westermeyer et al. (1991) report a suicide rate of approximately 9% in young people in the early phase of schizophrenia and suggest that the early phase of a psychotic illness (i.e., the first 6 years) may be a critical period for suicide to occur among individuals with schizophrenia and other psychotic disorders.

In summary, the experience of a first episode of psychosis is devastating emotionally for the individual and has the capacity to cause significant damage to a young person's sense of self, especially because it strikes at a time in development when identity formation is at the forefront. The emotional experiences encountered by young people recovering from their first episode of this illness may, at times, be so intense that hopelessness and depression ensue. These young people have significant barriers to overcome as they struggle to recover from their illness. Stigma and misconceptions associated with a diagnosis of schizophrenia are powerful influences that can significantly alter how the person views him- or herself and his or her future possibilities.

Impact of Early Schizophrenia on Self-Concept

It has been argued that what "individuals believe about themselves is more important than any other form of knowledge" (Strauman and Higgins 1993). Whether a person possesses a strong, coherent sense of self or a shaky, fragmented sense of self ultimately affects the individual's ability to overcome adversity (Segal and Blatt 1993). Chronic illness and its treatment challenge an individual's sense of who he or she is (Charmaz 1983, 1991). For young people encountering a first episode of schizophrenia, the question of what they will continue to believe about themselves is foremost. The self that they have known is immediately called into question as they realize that they have an illness that they themselves have previously identified as highly stigmatizing (Link 1987). Deegan (1993) described the profound problem of identifying with preconceived stigmatizing ideas about mental illness and schizophrenia, as exemplified by phrases such as "psychopathic killers" and "lunatics."

Society continues to hold highly stigmatized attitudes toward individuals with mental illness (Fink and Tasman 1992), such that individuals prefer to maintain considerable social distance from those whom they perceive to be mentally ill (Link 1987). Society's stigmatizing attitudes and behaviors are readily incorporated into the young person's identity (Beiser et al. 1987), resulting in negative attitudes toward diagnosis and treatment and, ultimately, negative self-concepts. Individuals with mental illness, especially those encountering the illness for the first time, may feel devalued, worthless, and socially undesirable.

As a result of these pervasive negative societal attitudes, individuals with schizophrenia are likely to actively withdraw from others to protect themselves from being rebuked and being the target of negative feedback. Based on clinical experience, young people with this illness talk about their fears of being judged and rejected by friends and family for having mental illness. In our group intervention, one young man recounted that he had taken a risk and called an old friend to see a movie with him. The group supported him in taking this courageous step and felt extremely saddened and outraged when this young man's friend openly refused the invitation and essentially ended the relationship. The group was able to discuss this and reached a consensus that acceptance of mental illness was the "acid test" of true friendship. Whether or not to disclose stigmatizing information presents a tremendous challenge for young people with early schizophrenia. For all individuals with a chronic illness, an awareness of being different and the ongoing internal debate about whether to reveal illness-related information can severely strain all relationships (Lubkin 1998).

Young people who participated in our group intervention all described a period of isolation and withdrawal after the psychotic episode. Gradual loss of social relationships and roles over time has been referred to as *progressive role constriction*, which may ultimately lead to the adoption of the chronic patient role (Estroff 1989). The fact that the onset of schizophrenia usually occurs in adolescence or early adulthood may contribute to the thoroughness and chronicity of role constriction because this is a time when roles are fluid, not yet stabilized, and vulnerable to change (Erikson 1968; Juhasz 1989). Lubkin (1998) discussed the process of social isolation in the chronically ill population in general. She observed that as the ill person becomes increasingly aware of the constricting network, he or she experiences emotions such as despair, sadness, anger, and loss of self-esteem, all of which contribute to changes in personal and social identity. Through this process of social withdrawal, "basic human needs for intimacy remain unmet" (Lubkin 1998, p. 184).

For some of the young people attending our group, it was even difficult to share illness-related information with family members. One young man was instructed by his parents not to disclose any information about his illness to anyone outside the family, including his extended family. This young man believed that he could not attend family functions for fear of not knowing what to say about his situation and inadvertently revealing his illness. A young woman in the group referred to herself as "damaged goods" and was afraid that she would never be able to marry or have any kind of intimate relationship in the future. Any opportunity for young people with this illness to openly discuss the stigma associated with mental illness and any negative responses that they have observed or experienced with clinicians or peers in a group setting serves to reduce the sense of isolation and provides a bridge to developing new relationships.

As a result of the profound stigma that continues to be associated with schizophrenia and the resultant social isolation, young people with this illness are vulnerable to the phenomenon of illness engulfment, whereby personal identity is lost. Individuals who are engulfed consider themselves as only exemplars of a particular "illness" (Estroff 1989; Lally 1989). Engulfment is a process in the chronic illness experience manifested by a loss of the sense of self, which results in the self-concept's being increasingly organized around the illness and around the patient role. Engulfment is manifested by alterations in self-concept and adoption of the illness role. Specifically, individuals who are engulfed by their illness experience a loss of normal roles, a sense of having been changed by the illness, and a loss of self-esteem (Lally 1989; McCay and Seeman 1998). Individuals engulfed by their illness usually accept the mental illness label and make negative comparisons of themselves to others (Lally 1989;

McCay and Seeman 1998). Overall, the changes that accompany engulfment are viewed as relatively permanent. Research evidence indicates
that engulfment in patients with schizophrenia is accompanied by hopelessness, depression, low self-esteem, a lack of self-efficacy, and decreased social adjustment (McCay 1994; McCay and Seeman 1998) and
may be a precursor to the development of the negative syndrome or the
descent into chronicity.

Individuals frequently feel damaged and engulfed by their illness. In
the extreme, young people with schizophrenia may view all future aspirations as untenable. Young people may also perceive that clinicians either implicitly or overtly agree that the illness has precluded any chance
of normal aspirations such as career and relationships. As is discussed in
the section of this chapter on intervention, strategies that convey to
young adults recovering from first-episode schizophrenia that they are
more than their illness—by inquiring about personal goals, interests,
likes, and dislikes—contribute to the reformulation of a healthier sense
of self. In this way, these young people may feel appreciated for who
they are as individuals, distinct from their illness, with potential and ca-
pabilities to resume previously held life goals. For instance, when asked
about her spring garden, a young woman very early in the course of treatment replied with much brighter affect that no one had asked her about
herself in such a long time.

Ultimately, a redefinition of the self is required for individuals recovering from first-episode schizophrenia (Albiston et al. 1998; Davidson and
Strauss 1992), one that incorporates and accommodates the illness in a
positive and realistic light yet resists the precarious risk of engulfment. It
may be true that a healthy sense of self will enable young people recovering from a first episode of schizophrenia to resist the engulfing effects
of the illness and to rebuild meaningful lives. Given the significance of
engulfment for clinical outcome and the adaptive potential of a strong
and coherent sense of self, it is imperative that these two clinical variables
be held uppermost in the clinician's mind as a guide to meeting the patient's emotional needs.

Intervention

The early phase of psychosis may offer important opportunities for secondary prevention (Birchwood et al. 1998; Jackson et al. 1996; McGorry
1992). It is becoming increasingly evident that the earliest possible instance in the illness trajectory is the most important time to focus on in-

terventions to enhance individuals' sense of self and self-efficacy to minimize the deleterious effects associated with entrenchment of negative self-views (Jackson et al. 1998). Growing evidence suggests there is a critical period of about 2–5 years after the onset of the disorder during which treatment has a maximal impact on outcome (Birchwood and Mac-Millan 1993; Birchwood et al. 1997). It may be possible, then, to influence the course of the disorder during this time and therefore to prevent further deterioration and engulfment of the person in the role of the chronic mental patient.

Individual Support

In recent years, there has been a shift away from intensive, interpretive individual psychotherapy for persons with schizophrenia toward more supportive approaches that focus primarily on adjustment to illness. The approaches described in this chapter are largely supportive; however, given the heterogeneous nature of the illness course and outcome in schizophrenia, it is important to tailor the approach to the individual. It is critical to consider the individual's vulnerability to relapse and the presence of any residual symptoms and cognitive deficits. Assessment of individuals should also include their capacity for introspection, ability to express themselves in words, and ability to tolerate frustration and unpleasant affect without reacting in a destructive manner. A supportive psychotherapy style that conveys an understanding and acceptance of the individual's subjective states (Wasylenki 1992) is particularly effective with individuals who demonstrate an interest in addressing other issues, such as preexisting problems in personality and functioning, after the psychosis has resolved (Greenfeld 1985).

Intervention strategies that address the person's emotional response to a first episode of psychosis, including the meaning of the illness experience, are critical to alleviate emotional suffering and to enable the patient to cope with and survive the illness experience. The adjustment process to a first episode of psychosis can be viewed as involving a search for the meaning in the experience, an attempt to regain mastery over the event and over one's life more generally, and an effort to restore self-esteem through self-enhancing evaluations (Jackson et al. 1996; McGorry 1992, 1995). The establishment of a supportive, consistent therapeutic relationship during recovery is necessary to assist the person in this endeavor and to facilitate adjustment to the illness without despair. As individuals recover from a psychotic episode, they often feel frightened, alone, and deeply ashamed as they begin to realize they are suffering from a highly stigmatizing illness. A therapeutic relationship can provide comfort and acceptance, particularly through understanding of the person's subjective experience. Self-psychology theory (Baker and Baker 1987), with its focus on empathic listening, understanding, and affirmation of the person's sense of self, offers a framework for clinicians to achieve understanding of the person's subjective experience and to enhance the person's sense of self.

In our experience, many young people recovering from a first episode of psychosis benefit from an opportunity to talk about the illness experience and make some sense of it as they struggle to come to terms with the illness. The process of talking with patients about the actual experience of illness and helping to order and make sense of that experience may have therapeutic value (Kleinman 1988). Sharing painful feelings related to the episode (e.g., shame, sadness, and alienation) with a therapist often provides relief and a sense of feeling understood and accepted. Eliciting and understanding patients' interpretations and explanatory models of illness (Kleinman 1988) are important aspects of this process. Many people have personal ideas about how their illness came about and how it is to be dealt with. Some may feel they are to blame for the illness. Others may not view themselves as having suffered an illness. How persons view their illness and their vulnerability to relapse influence their acceptance of the need for ongoing treatment and, in turn, their long-term adjustment. Exploring illness meanings and explanatory models elucidates important issues to address, including potential barriers to treatment. Additionally, it provides opportunities to correct negative and damaging misconceptions about the illness.

There are some individuals with whom this may not be a suitable approach, at least in the initial phases of the illness. For example, individuals who continue to experience psychotic symptoms, profound negative symptoms, or cognitive deficits may not be ready or able to talk about the illness experience and its impact. These individuals may benefit more from structured psychosocial rehabilitation programs that focus on coping skills and a gradual step-by-step approach to resuming tasks and activities. Additionally, individuals who deny their illness or who are not in touch with their feelings about their situation may not be ready to engage in the process of talking about the illness experience. For these individuals, establishing a therapeutic relationship is often very challenging and requires much flexibility, patience, and persistence on the part of the therapist. Rather than emphasizing the experience of illness, the clinician may need to "hang in" with these individuals to facilitate the development of a therapeutic alliance by being available to help with practical issues identified by the individual, such as housing or finances. Some evidence suggests that the establishment of a therapeutic alliance within the first 6 months of treatment may be critical to engagement in therapy, adherence to medication, and better outcomes (Frank and Gunderson 1990). In our experience, it is critical to begin working on an alliance as soon as possible, ideally while the person is in the hospital, to provide continuity in care and facilitate adherence to outpatient follow-up. It is also essential to start with "where the patient is at" and pace yourself accordingly.

One young woman experiencing hostility and paranoid ideation adamantly denied her illness and saw no need for antipsychotic medication. The chances of engaging her in ongoing supportive therapy seemed slim. However, through the clinician's "being there," listening, and offering support and compassion, she eventually came to trust her clinician. Over the course of a few years, she became more compliant with her medication treatment. She did eventually talk about her experience of psychosis and her difficulties accepting the diagnosis of schizophrenia. Although she never fully acknowledged having a mental illness, she did understand that she had some difficulties for which she required assistance from a mental health professional. Another patient, a young man, had been ill for several years and recently began treatment. When asked why he did not come for treatment sooner, he replied that he feared being labeled with a mental illness and then being stigmatized by society. An awareness on the part of the clinician of just how difficult and painful it is for many individuals to come to terms with the illness can provide a more sensitive, less pejorative understanding of the patient's denial of illness and noncompliance with treatment.

As mentioned, coping with stigma is perhaps one of the most difficult and painful challenges these young people must face. It is often helpful and empowering for individuals to recognize that stigma reflects others' personal difficulties and lack of knowledge and awareness regarding mental illness. Recognizing that other people also have limitations—in others words, that nobody is perfect—is also a helpful coping strategy. Providing opportunities for contact with others who have been through a similar illness is a potent source of support for these young people and helps to counteract stigma.

In an effort to cope with feelings of low self-esteem and engulfment, individuals frequently voice the importance of trying to move beyond the illness and get on with their lives. There seems to be a growing sense of hope as individuals distance themselves from the illness and become re-acquainted with themselves. The clinician can facilitate this process by actively striving to help individuals reconnect with aspects of themselves that are unrelated to illness. It is often helpful for clinicians to encourage individuals to contemplate who they were before the onset of the illness. By drawing on individuals' personal interests, values, or beliefs, the therapist communicates to them that the therapist sees them as individuals with potential and strengths and, most importantly, that they are more than an illness. This strategy may contribute to an enhanced sense of self beyond the illness, instill hope, and open up possibilities for the future. In addition, the development of an enhanced sense of self provides the person with resources to battle negative forces in the environment, such as stigma (Davidson and Strauss 1992). Hope seems to play a critical role in the recovery process and in the development of an enhanced sense of self. Time and time again, our clinical work has highlighted the importance of the clinician's having hope, not giving up, and keeping an open mind about what is possible. Similarly, in a study of sense of self and recovery from prolonged and severe mental illness, Davidson and Strauss (1992) found that persons who improved often gave some credit for an awakening of hope to important people in their lives who believed in them or had faith in them.

The critical role of hope is illustrated by another young woman who suffered from schizophrenia and was constantly tortured by critical, derogatory auditory hallucinations. She had lost all confidence in herself and felt completely at the mercy of her voices. She was incapacitated by her illness and was unable to carry out even the most basic of activities of daily living. She felt that she could not do anything on her own and required much support from her mother. Although she was quite demoralized and despondent at times, she never entirely gave up hope that someday she might resume her studies in psychology. Therapy focused on helping her take small steps toward independence (e.g., coming to appointments eventually on her own), highlighting the smallest steps and signs of progress (e.g., cooking a meal for herself or walking to the corner store on her own), and exploring and encouraging efforts to cope with the voices. There was also much discussion about her future aspirations, which seemed to give her tremendous strength to carry on day to day and brought meaning to her life. Over the course of 5 years, she gradually gained more confidence, felt empowered, and achieved a sense of mastery over the illness. She was eventually able to resume her studies on a part-time basis.

Psychoeducation

Education about the illness can provide a framework for understanding and making sense of the illness experience (explanatory model), correcting negative misconceptions and stereotypes associated with schizophrenia, and promoting a sense of mastery. It also has the potential to instill hope and facilitate engagement in treatment (McGorry 1995).

However, our clinical experience suggests that information about the illness and diagnosis may contribute to feelings of demoralization and hopelessness, sometimes alienating patients from the very support they need. Most individuals react strongly to hearing the diagnosis of schizophrenia. We believe this is because of the negative stereotypes and stigma associated with the label of schizophrenia, as well as the pessimism expressed in the literature about recovery and outcome. For this reason, illness-related information needs to be conveyed in a sensitive manner, and the rate at which the information is provided also needs to be considered. In addition, patients' reactions to the information should be carefully monitored. For example, one young woman felt that being told she has schizophrenia was similar to "being given a life sentence." Another said it was similar to being told she has cancer, with no hope for recovery. Thus, education about the illness and its implications requires attention to such illness meanings and sensitivity to the person's need for time to work through and resolve the illness experience. It is critical that the therapist actively encourage optimism about outcome and correct negative misconceptions. It should also be emphasized that everyone's experience of psychosis is different and that the illness course and outcome vary from person to person. In addition, psychoeducation with this patient population requires sensitivity to diagnostic complexity and uncertainty (McGorry 1995) because some individuals who experience a first episode of schizophrenia may not remain diagnostically stable.

Persons recovering from a first episode of schizophrenia need to understand that there is a risk of relapse. The vulnerability model of illness (Zubin and Spring 1977) encompasses the notion of biological vulnerability and the role of psychosocial factors and stress in precipitating onset and influencing the course of illness. The vulnerability model of illness is a helpful framework for understanding the illness and encourages an active role for the person in the prevention of relapse. There are a number of steps the person can take to stay well, such as taking medication, learning about early warning signs of the illness, using stress management techniques, building up a support network, and engaging in valued activities such as work, school, or leisure. Individuals often need encouragement to resume school or work gradually during the recovery period to minimize stress. Taking an active role in treatment and recovery and knowing that there are strategies that can be taken to facilitate recovery and prevent relapse can be very empowering.

Research Studies

There have been few specialized studies of individual psychological interventions for persons recovering from a first episode of psychosis. Jackson et al. (1996, 1998) have now described a cognitively oriented psychotherapy for early psychosis (COPE). Their approach uses psychoeducation and cognitive techniques to challenge self-stigmatization, help the person come to terms with understanding their illness, and help the patient pursue life goals. The overall strategy is aimed at helping the person adjust to the illness without despair. The self and the person's response to the disorder is a key focus. The goals of therapy are to 1) assist the person in a search for the meaning in the experience; 2) promote a sense of mastery over the experience; and 3) to protect and enhance self-esteem, which has been severely threatened or damaged by the onset of the disorder. As in our approach, the COPE model integrates an exploration of the person's explanatory model of illness and the gentle nurturing of that model, which facilitates optimal participation in treatment without damaging the person (Jackson et al. 1998). Preliminary pilot results suggest that this approach may be promising; however, the results need to be replicated in a randomized controlled trial (Jackson et al. 1998).

As previously described, the authors have developed a focused, module-based group intervention to address psychological adjustment to illness in the first-episode population. Peer groups play a central role during the transition from adolescence to adulthood. Thus, the group setting can provide young adults with schizophrenia an opportunity to construct a positive self-concept through interacting with others, exploring the meaning of illness, developing an acceptable understanding of the illness, and developing ways of coping with distressing symptoms. The overall goal of the group developed from our pilot group (McCay et al. 1996) and is to encourage participants to resist engulfment through exploring illness meanings and reactions, alleviating alienation, augmenting coping skills, working out a positive identity in the context of illness, and engendering a view of the future that encompasses the retention of possibilities.

An evaluation study is currently being completed. At present, a within-group analysis of 29 group subjects who have participated in one of five group trials indicates that participants experience significantly decreased engulfment, hopelessness, symptoms, and emotion-based coping at the 3-month follow-up evaluation compared with the preintervention evaluation. Qualitative data analysis of the group transcripts illustrates the goals of the group and that group members were actively engaged in the group.

The themes of working through and making sense of the illness were viewed as especially important by the individuals who participated in the group intervention. Participants also described the struggle to preserve a sense of self that is separate from the illness. Group members reported that receiving support and understanding from others who have had similar experiences was a valuable and unique experience. It was striking that participants were both surprised and impressed that other group members had similar illness experiences and emotional responses to these experiences. The group members' sense of surprise seemed to suggest that members were reassured to find other pleasant, articulate young people at the group, rather than individuals who appeared to have been ravaged by years of chronic mental illness. Recognition of group members' mutual strengths seemed to convey "if you appear all right to me, then I must appear all right to you and others beyond the group." Accordingly, the discussion in the group also emphasized the critical role of stigma for young adults attempting to deal with early schizophrenia. Despite feeling negatively about the diagnosis of schizophrenia, participants were able to identify that they possessed a vulnerability to symptoms or difficulties that interfered with functioning and required treatment.

In summary, psychological interventions play a critical role in the adjustment process to a first episode of schizophrenia and may prevent secondary impairments, including damage to the person's sense of self. Deegan (1993) emphasized that no one (professional or nonprofessional) addressed with her the fact that her identity was stripped away from her or acknowledged the profound depths of her psychological suffering after her first episode. Deegan and members of our group assert that it is possible to recover from the effects of being labeled as schizophrenic and the trauma of hospitalization and to rebuild a meaningful life.

Outcome

Outcome is a critically important concept that needs to be considered specifically in the context of first-episode schizophrenia. What the young person with newly diagnosed schizophrenia believes about outcome and the promise of what life may hold affects all aspects of psychological adjustment. It is a significant challenge for individuals with first-episode schizophrenia to hold on to a sense of an optimistic future or destiny after their life trajectory is altered by the onset of this illness. A young person with schizophrenia is frequently assumed to be destined for a severely compromised life that is bereft of life-sustaining forces such as a satisfying occupation and companionship. This negative view of schizophrenia has been in existence since the time of Kraepelin (McGorry 1998), who identified schizophrenia as a progressively deteriorating disease. Treatment settings frequently bring young people with a first episode of schizophrenia into contact with individuals who have been treated for long periods of time and have been disabled by the illness. Young people in our clinical practice have found that encountering individuals who had been ill for some time raised questions about whether their own futures would be reflective of chronic mental illness. One young man used the words "there goes my future" when describing his reactions to individuals with chronic schizophrenia, and a young woman was constantly preoccupied with fears of becoming a "bag lady."

Recent scientific advances in understanding the biochemical mechanisms underlying schizophrenia have enabled the development of much more effective pharmacotherapy (Remington et al. 1998) to treat the illness. At this time in the treatment of patients with schizophrenia, an increased sense of hope is beginning to develop with regard to the potential of young people to achieve satisfying and fulfilling lives. This renewed hope needs to be communicated to today's generation of young people who are struggling with the preconceived negative expectations surrounding schizophrenia. A direct attempt to communicate the belief that young people with schizophrenia can continue to work toward life goals can significantly heighten the individual's and family's expectation for improved outcome and could help to avoid a legacy of chronicity and despair.

Within the context of the literature that addresses the impact of psychological adjustment on outcome overall, it is important to consider what constitutes a meaningful outcome for young adults recovering from a first episode of schizophrenia. Hatfield and Lefley (1993) offer a salient perspective, suggesting that recovery is not necessarily synonymous with the absence of symptoms or complete return of functioning; rather, recovery is a "process of adaptation at increasingly higher levels of personal satisfaction and interpersonal functioning. It involves finding meaning and purpose to life that goes beyond the limitations imposed by the disorder" (p. 41). Anthony (1993) suggested that, in many instances, emotional expression (e.g., depression, guilt, and isolation) is too frequently considered as part of the illness and not part of the recovery process. Anthony argued that attention to the emotional needs of patients is part of a larger recovery vision that enables individuals to go beyond the limitations imposed by their illness by living a vital, satisfying, and contributing life. Given the fact that functional levels have been found to be unrelated to symptoms (Birchwood et al. 1998), it is conceivable that personal satisfaction with life could be achieved despite unresolved symptoms. Crucial aspects of recovery and outcome not only need to include symptom reduction and the occurrence of relapse but also additional variables such as self-esteem, self-determination, adjustment to disability (Anthony 1993), and the capacity to move beyond the illness to pursue satisfying activities, interests, and relationships. As young people recover from a first episode of schizophrenia, it is not unusual for them to describe their illness as a growth experience because they have achieved a level of maturity far beyond their years. They describe knowing human suffering, how to grow beyond suffering and disregard the trivial, and to embrace what is important in life.

Although no conclusive research studies substantiate the impact of emotional needs on outcome, the literature is replete with descriptive studies and observations that suggest that failing to effectively address the emotional needs of those recovering from early schizophrenia may further induce emotional trauma and, over time, may fuel the downward spiral of chronicity. The most dramatic outcome that may be linked to a failure to meet the emotional needs of patients is the high rate of suicide in early schizophrenia. As mentioned, the suicide rate has been reported to be 9% in the earliest phase of a schizophrenic illness (Westermeyer et al. 1991). Birchwood et al. (1998) reviewed the literature related to suicide in early schizophrenia and concluded that psychological factors, such as a fear of the deteriorating effects of the illness, a sense of failed expectations, and an underlying sense of hopelessness, are the most potent contributors to suicide completion rather than psychotic thinking as frequently assumed. Denial and chronic depression were also identified as psychological factors that, if not addressed, may exacerbate early decline. Specifically, denial jeopardizes optimal outcome through increased risk of suicide and lack of adherence to prescribed treatment. In addition, sustained depression is associated with perceived lack of illness control and the assumption of negative stereotypes, consistent with

McCay and Seeman's (1998) findings related to the engulfing effects of schizophrenia.

It is readily acknowledged by several authors that optimal management, including psychosocial interventions, is required to achieve full recovery (Power et al. 1998; Wyatt et al. 1998). The time immediately after the initial episode of schizophrenia is also thought to be the ideal time to prevent secondary psychological impairments that have significant impact on long-term outcome (Birchwood et al. 1998). Two illustrative psychological interventions that help individuals adjust to their illness without despair have been described. One intervention is the COPE program (Jackson et al. 1998), which is designed to challenge self-stigmatization and facilitate the recovery process, and the other one is an innovative group intervention (McCay et al. 1996) that enables young people to work out a positive identity in the context of their illness and to embrace an optimistic view of the future. Both the COPE program and our group intervention program illustrate the critical role that psychological interventions assume in achieving optimal outcome and well being in patients with first-episode schizophrenia.

Evidence from studies on patients with chronic schizophrenia also indicates that psychosocial interventions are most likely important treatments that may not only enhance the psychological adjustment to the illness but also have the potential to reduce relapse rates in first-episode schizophrenia (Falloon et al. 1998; Wyatt et al. 1998). Despite the documented role that psychosocial interventions assume in achieving optimal outcome, the difficult question remains of what specific psychological interventions contribute to enhanced outcome for those recovering from first-episode schizophrenia.

Conclusions

Responding to the emotional needs of individuals recovering from first-episode schizophrenia is challenging yet highly rewarding clinical work. Given the expectations for improved outcomes in first-episode illness, opportunities exist for clinicians to influence the course of the schizophrenia illness trajectory. Supportive clinical interventions planned according to the needs and strengths of the individual within the context of a consistent therapeutic relationship can effectively facilitate the patient's ability to surmount the many challenges to illness adaptation. Given individuals' fears of stigmatization and rejection, it is crucial that the clinician convey an attitude of nonjudgmental acceptance as well as a willingness to work through patients' illness experience. As part of trying to make sense of the illness experience, the clinician can expect and encourage the expression of illness-related feelings such as shame, sadness, fear, anger, and alienation. In addition, patients usually bring very strong negative associations to the illness and, as described, experience very real instances of stigma and rejection. It is not at all surprising or unrealistic that patients actively resist the diagnosis of schizophrenia. Clinicians need to be willing to discuss patients' questions and resistance to the diagnosis and to consider alternate explanatory illness models. Through these dialogues, patients become aware that the clinician is not trying to label them with society's negative perceptions of schizophrenia but that, instead, the clinician is genuinely interested in helping them to gain control of the illness and to reclaim their lives.

The formation of a working alliance and movement toward acceptance of the illness can take considerable time. Ongoing patience and encouragement from the clinician, despite expressions of denial and noncompliance with treatment, can help patients to negotiate the painful journey of coming to terms with the illness. To move toward illness acceptance, it is helpful for patients to realize that stigma reflects a general lack of knowledge and understanding about mental illness and is in no way a reflection of themselves or the illness. To actively counter the stigma and the negative expectations of future outcomes usually associated with schizophrenia, the clinician needs to assert that it is possible to work toward life goals. Clinicians can also reduce the risk of engulfment by the illness by actively promoting a strong and coherent sense of self. An explicit interest in the patient as a person, including his or her likes, dislikes, interests, and ambitions, conveys to the patient that the clinician does not see them as just schizophrenic but rather as a whole individual who has the potential to resume their life goals. Promoting patients' active involvement in treatment and recovery through opportunities to learn about strategies for managing the illness is another effective vehicle to promote a healthy, competent sense of self. In particular, encouraging patients to become familiar with the role of stress in precipitating relapse is an effective mechanism for developing a sense of control over the illness.

Although no conclusive research studies substantiate the impact of emotional adjustment on outcome, it is increasingly evident that meeting the emotional needs of patients must form the foundation for treatment so individuals may overcome the psychological trauma associated with the illness by engaging in health-promoting strategies that maximize their potential to lead satisfying and rewarding lives. Although adjustment to a first episode of schizophrenia poses an extraordinary challenge for all involved (i.e., individuals, families, and health care professionals), there is no question that surmounting the adversity surrounding the illness is possible and may be anticipated, as reflected in this quote from one young man in recovery:

> Everyone has challenges in their lives and this is just another significant challenge to overcome. Your strength of character really has a lot to do with how successful you're going to be in overcoming the illness. You see a hurdle in front of you and you may try to jump over it, and you can't cross the hurdle...Or you can do the alternative and keep trying and keep trying to jump over it, and continue with your life. And I think that's been a more positive way of viewing this entire situation.

References

Addington D, Addington J, Patten S: Depression in people with first-episode schizophrenia. Br J Psychiatry 172(suppl 33):90–92, 1998

Albiston DJ, Francey SM, Harrigan SM: Group programs for recovery from early psychosis. Br J Psychiatry 172(suppl 33):117–121, 1998

Anthony W: Recovery from mental illness: the guiding vision of the mental health service system. Psychosocial Rehabilitation Journal 16:11–23, 1993

Baker HS, Baker MN: Heinz Kohut's self psychology: an overview. Am J Psychiatry 144:1–9, 1987

Beiser M, Waler-Morrison N, Aachen WG, et al: A measure of the "sick" label in psychiatric disorder and physical illness. Soc Sci Med 25:251–261, 1987

Birchwood M, MacMillan F: Early intervention in schizophrenia. Aust NZ J Psychiatry 27:374–378, 1993

Birchwood M, McGorry P, Jackson H: Early intervention in schizophrenia. Br J Psychiatry 170:2–5, 1997

Birchwood M, Todd P, Jackson C: Early intervention in psychosis. Br J Psychiatry 172(suppl 33):53–59, 1998

Charmaz K: Loss of self: a fundamental form of suffering in the chronically ill. Sociology of Health and Illness 5:168–195, 1983

Charmaz K: Good Days, Bad Days: The Self in Chronic Illness and Time. New Brunswick, NJ, Rutgers University Press, 1991

Davidson L, Strauss JS: Sense of self in recovery from severe mental illness. Br J Med Psychol 65:131–145, 1992

Deegan PE: Recovering our sense of being labeled. J Psychosoc Nurs 31:7–11, 1993

Drake RE, Sederer LI: Inpatient psychosocial treatment of chronic schizophrenia: negative effects and current guidelines. Hospital and Community Psychiatry 37:897–901, 1986

Erikson EL: Youth and Crisis. New York, Norton, 1968

Estroff SE: Self, identity, and subjective experiences of schizophrenia: in search of the subject. Schizophr Bull 15:189–196, 1989

Falloon I, Coverdale J, Laidlaw T, et al: Early intervention for schizophrenic disorders. Br J Psychiatry 172(suppl 33):33–38, 1998

Fink PJ, Tasman A: Stigma and mental Illness. Washington, DC, American Psychiatric Press, 1992

Frank AF, Gunderson, JG: The role of the treatment alliance in the treatment of schizophrenia. Arch Gen Psychiatry 47:228–236, 1990

Greenfeld D: The Psychotic Patient: Medication and Psychotherapy. New York, The Free Press, 1985

Hatfield A, Lefley H: Surviving Mental Illness: Stress, Coping and Adaptation. New York, Guilford, 1993

Jackson H, McGorry P, Edwards J, et al: Cognitively oriented psychotherapy in early psychosis—COPE, in Early Intervention and Prevention in Mental Health. Edited by Cotton PJ, Jackson HJ. Melbourne, Australia, Australian Psychological Society, 1996, pp 131–154

Jackson H, McGorry P, Edwards J, et al: Cognitively oriented psychotherapy for early psychosis (COPE). Br J Psychiatry 172(suppl 33):93–100, 1998

Juhasz A: A role based approach to adult development: the triple helix model. Int J Aging Hum Devel 29:301–315, 1989

Kleinman A: Illness meanings and illness behavior, in Illness Behavior: A Multidisciplinary Approach. Edited by McHugh S, Valis T. New York, Plenum, 1988, pp 149–160

Koreen AR, Siris SG, Chakos M, et al: Depression in first-episode schizophrenia. Am J Psychiatry 150:1643–1648, 1993

Lally SJ: "Does being in here mean there is something wrong with me?" Schizophr Bull 15:253–265, 1989

Link BG: Understanding labeling effects in the area of mental disorders: an assessment of the effects of expectations of rejection. Am Sociol Rev 52:96–112, 1987

Lubkin I: Chronic Illness: Impact and Interventions. Toronto, Canada, Jones and Bartlett, 1998

McCay E: The Construct Validation of the Modified Engulfment Scale. Unpublished doctoral dissertation. University of Toronto, Toronto, Canada, 1994

McCay E, Seeman M: A scale to measure the impact of a schizophrenic illness on an individual's self-concept. Arch Psychiatr Nurs 12:41–49, 1998

McCay E, Ryan K, Amey S: Mitigating engulfment: recovering from a first episode of psychosis. J Psychosoc Nurs 34:40–44, 1996

McGlashen TH, Carpenter WT: Postpsychotic depression in schizophrenia. Arch Gen Psychiatry 33:231–239, 1976

McGorry P: The concept of recovery and secondary prevention in psychotic disorders. Aust NZ J Psychiatry 237:3–17, 1992

McGorry P: Psychoeducation in first-episode psychosis: a therapeutic process. Psychiatry 58:313–328, 1995

McGorry P: Preventive strategies in early psychosis: verging on reality. Br J Psychiatry 172(suppl 33):93–100, 1998

McGorry PD, Chanen A, McCarthy E, et al: Posttraumatic stress disorder following recent-onset psychosis: an unrecognized post-psychotic syndrome. J Nerv Ment Dis 17:253–258, 1991

Plasky P: Antidepressant usage in schizophrenia. Schizophr Bull 17:649–657, 1991

Power P, Elkins K, Adard S, et al: Analysis of the initial treatment phase in first episode psychosis. Br J Psychiatry 172(suppl 33):71–76, 1998

Remington G, Kapur S, Zipursky RB: Pharmacotherapy of first episode schizophrenia. Br J Psychiatry 172(suppl):66–70, 1998

Segal Z, Blatt S: The Self in Emotional Distress: Cognitive and Psychodynamic Perspectives. New York, Guilford, 1993

Strauman T, Higgins E: The self construct in social cognitions: past, present, and future, in The Self in Emotional Distress: Cognitive and Psychodynamic Perspectives. Edited by Segal Z, Blatt S. New York, Guilford, 1993, pp 3–40

Wasylenki D: Psychotherapy of schizophrenia revisited. Hospital and Community Psychiatry 43:123–127, 1992

Westermeyer JF, Harrow M, Marengo JT: Risk for suicide in schizophrenia and other psychotic and nonpsychotic disorders. J Nerv Ment Dis 179:259–266, 1991

Wyatt R, Damiani L, Henter I: First episode schizophrenia. Br J Psychiatry 172(suppl 33):77–83, 1998

Zubin J, Spring B: Vulnerability: a new view of schizophrenia. J Abnorm Psychol 86:102–126, 1977

Family Intervention in the Early Stages of Schizophrenia

April A. Collins, M.S.W.

Schizophrenia is a disorder that has been recognized in almost all cultures and has been described through much of recorded time (Black and Andreasen 1994). Remarkably, despite being the focus of research for decades, it remains one of the most enigmatic and devastating of the psychiatric disorders (Kay 1990). Current estimates suggest that approximately 20%–30% of those diagnosed with schizophrenia are able to lead somewhat normal lives, 20%–30% continue to experience moderate difficulties, and 40%–60% are left significantly impaired for extended periods of time (Breier et al. 1991). Consequently, for most patients, the onset of schizophrenia is not simply a short-term crisis that resolves and goes away. Rather, it is the beginning of a complex set of changing issues with a history and a future course (Rutter 1987).

Currently, few systematic studies describe the effect of first-episode psychosis on families or their needs in dealing with such an illness. Consequently, when clinicians are working with these new families, they remain dependent on and tend to use the knowledge generated by studies that examine family intervention in chronic schizophrenia. It is common, for example, to hear families being encouraged to read literature on "surviving schizophrenia" and to participate in groups that typically focus on coping with very debilitating and protracted forms of the illness. From a clinical standpoint, there is reason to question the appropriateness and utility of these approaches for families with members who have experienced first episodes of schizophrenia. The onset of psychosis in a child can precipitate some of the deepest anguish that parents are likely to experience, and this usually affects every aspect of family life. Coming to terms with the illness can be a demanding, painful, and slow process, one that should not be rushed by clinicians in their desire to have families accept the diagnosis. Initially, partial denial of the threat of illness through disbelief, nonacceptance, or avoidance may be adaptive and often helps parents deal with the unknowns associated with the illness at a manageable pace rather than being overwhelmed by catastrophic possibilities. Parents are repeatedly confronted by the competing forces of reality and desire for homeostasis. The former demands that they experience the painful realization of their potential loss, and the latter requires that they seek sanctuary from this painful realization. Ideally, our goal is to help families achieve a balance between the demands of reality and the safety provided by mechanisms that tend to obfuscate reality (Zisook 1987). When people are completely stripped of their defenses (i.e., by reading information on chronic schizophrenia during a first episode), they are left feeling overwhelmed and paralyzed. From a clinical standpoint, we must recognize the importance of timing in all of our work; in this way, we can help parents focus on current issues with respect to their child's illness and "dose" any of the pain associated with the problems that arise.

This chapter begins with a brief review of the history of family intervention in schizophrenia and the origins of the construct of expressed emotion (EE) and summarizes the results of the psychoeducational literature. This is followed by a discussion of finding new ways of viewing families that will allow us to move beyond the limitations of the previous era (Cook et al. 1997). Just as the idea of early detection and intervention at the first episode has raised the intriguing possibility of improving the natural course of schizophrenia for patients (Birchwood and Macmillan 1993; McGlashan 1998), the notion of intervention with families during a first episode of schizophrenia is also compelling because it may offer important opportunities for secondary prevention—that is, early family intervention may allow us to begin to ask questions about what underlies successful family adaptation after the advent of this illness. This, in turn, may help to identify and foster key processes that enable families to successfully navigate through the crises and prolonged hardship that schizophrenia has been known to impose.

Historical Perspectives

Solomon (1998) insightfully noted that a society's assumptions about severe mental illness influence the way families are treated. Belief systems surrounding mental illness determine whether relatives are informed about the illness, its course, and its treatment; whether they are included in the treatment process; and whether any provision is made to address the stress associated with the caregiving role (Solomon 1998). The power and influence of the dominant paradigm is readily apparent when one traces the history of interventions for families affected by schizophrenia. In the era before the discovery of antipsychotic agents and deinstitutionalization, it was routinely believed that families had a causal role in the development of schizophrenia. The long association between the observed disturbances in relationships in families in which a member had been diagnosed led to the premature conclusion that these disturbances preceded the onset of the illness and, in fact, contributed to it. The hypothesis implicating families as causal agents has its roots in the psychoanalytic movement that was dominant in the first half of the twentieth century. Consequently, a number of elaborate and colorful theories emerged, ranging from the notion of a schizophrenogenic mother who drove her children into the frightening world of psychosis (Fromm-Reichmann 1948) to that of poor interpersonal communication patterns, which resulted in "double-binds" for children and eventually caused symptoms to develop (Bateson et al. 1956). Undoubtedly, these approaches to understanding schizophrenia pitted professionals against families and pressured families to accept blame.

Fortunately, mainstream psychiatry's commitment to these theories has disappeared. Evidence supporting a genetic component of schizophrenia, accompanied by the introduction of antipsychotic agents and the poor results of analytically oriented family therapy, has facilitated this process (Bellack and Mueser 1993). Old psychogenic models have been abandoned and long since replaced with the vulnerability–stress model of schizophrenia (Zubin and Spring 1977). In keeping with this framework, the vicissitudes of schizophrenia are seen as being determined by the nature of the vulnerability and stress on the one hand and of the individual strengths and environmental supports on the other (McGlashan 1994). Thus, the onset, course, and ultimate outcome are seen as intricately and temporally bound to the complex interplay between biological and environmental factors (Ciompi 1988; Strauss et al. 1985; Zubin and Spring 1977). The list of specific vulnerabilities is extensive; a few have been demonstrated and many more postulated (Nuechterlein and Dawson 1984).

No discussion of the vulnerability–stress model would be complete without acknowledging the contextual factors that helped solidify this new perspective within the field of psychiatry. As data began to accumulate supporting genetic factors and neurochemical dysfunction in schizophrenia (Syvalanti 1994), corresponding successes in treating psychotic symptoms with neuroleptic agents also occurred. These breakthroughs prompted a shift within psychiatry, and the treatment of patients with schizophrenia was moved from within institutions out into the community. Consequently, partially remitted patients were discharged, and the responsibility for care was shifted from the state onto relatives (Goldstein and Miklowitz 1995). Maintenance antipsychotic medications were quickly established as the foundation of treatment for patients with schizophrenia; however, the protection afforded by them alone was only partial (Falloon et al. 1990; Johnson 1976; Leff and Wing 1971). For example, Hogarty et al. (1986) reported that whereas the mean relapse rate for patients after 1 year of continuous treatment with antipsychotic agents was 41%, those in a placebo condition had a relapse rate of 68%. Although medications offered some prophylaxis against decompensation, these results clearly offered support for the contention that environmental stressors exert considerable influence, even when patients are taking optimal doses (Falloon et al. 1984). Seemingly, it was both the deinstitutionalization movement, with the revolving-door phenomenon of frequent—but brief—hospitalizations, and the return of symptoms after remission had been achieved with neuroleptic agents that prompted many to vigorously pursue research questions related to the reciprocal influences between patients with schizophrenia and their environments. To date, systematic research on nonbiological environmental factors exists in only a few areas. Within this domain, stressful life events (Lukoff et al. 1984; Nuechterlein et al. 1992) and the construct of EE have been investigated as precipitants of symptomatic relapse.

Expressed Emotion

The notion that family relationships may be one of the more powerful environmental influences that shape the course and outcome of schizophrenia has its roots in English social psychiatry (Hooley 1985). It was there, approximately 40 years ago, that interest in delineating the factors within the family environment that increase the likelihood of relapse was born. The initial observational work by Brown (1959) and Brown et al. (1958) served as a catalyst for this line of investigation. It was this group that retrospectively reported that success or failure in the community after hospital discharge was associated with the type of living situation to which a person returned. Specifically, they found that patients who returned to live in large hostels or with family had increased rates of relapse compared with those returning to other types of housing. They further noted, in a later investigation, that patients returning to "high emotional involvement homes" were significantly more likely to relapse with florid psychotic symptoms during a 1-year follow-up period (Brown et al. 1962).

Throughout the late 1960s, these earliest descriptions were used and eventually transformed by Brown and Rutter (1966) into the original version of the Camberwell Family Interview (CFI) Schedule, which served as the first measure of EE. In their now classic replication, Brown et al. (1972) enrolled persons with a possible or probable diagnosis of schizophrenia and reported a significant association between the amount of EE shown by relatives at the time of the key admission and symptomatic relapse during the 9 months after discharge.

Vaughn and Leff (1976), in further examining the construct of EE, revised the initial version of the CFI for use in a series of now seminal studies and were again able to document support for the contention that high levels of criticism, hostility, and emotional overinvolvement were associated with an increased risk of relapse in the 9 months after discharge from a hospital (Vaughn and Leff 1976; Vaughn et al. 1984). In the past two decades, the EE construct has been extensively studied (Kavanagh 1992; Kuipers 1994). Since the earliest work, more than 30 studies in many countries have investigated the EE–relapse relationship in patients with schizophrenia.

EE is a powerful concept in schizophrenia research and has become regarded as an operationalized measure of environmental stress (Freeman 1989). However, this work does have critics. Despite the numerous replications, the use of the construct is still being aggressively debated (Bellack and Mueser 1993). Several concerns have been raised, including the fact that not all studies have established a link between high EE and relapse (Dulz and Hand 1986; Hogarty et al. 1988; Parker et al. 1988). In addition, the predictive use of EE is questionable for women (Hogarty 1985; Vaughn and Leff 1976; Vaughn et al. 1984, 1992) and first-episode patients (Barrelet et al. 1990; MacMillan et al. 1986a, 1986b; Nuechterlein et al. 1992; Stirling et al. 1993). The level of EE has at times been found to be a function of the severity of symptoms (Glynn et al. 1990; Strachan et al. 1986), and compliance with prescribed treatment appears to reduce the predictive value of EE (Vaughn and Leff 1976; Vaughn et al. 1984, 1992). It is not surprising, under the circumstances, to find researchers and clinicians still asking if EE is epiphenomenal to relapse. In other words, is the link between EE and relapse mediated by some other factor?

In an attempt to more fully address the predictive validity of EE and to put this debate to rest, a recent meta-analysis (Butzlaff and Hooley 1998) combined the findings of 27 studies to provide an estimate of the effect size associated with the EE–relapse relationship. Several significant results emerged. These investigators found that the mean effect size was $r=0.30$, thus confirming that EE is a small but statistically significant predictor of relapse in schizophrenia. They also found that although EE predicted relapse regardless of the chronicity of the illness, the magnitude of this relationship was strongest for patients with more severe forms of schizophrenia (Butzlaff and Hooley 1998). Additionally, although the EE construct is most closely aligned with research in schizophrenia, the mean effect sizes for both mood disorders ($r=0.39$) and eating disorders ($r=0.51$) were significantly higher than the mean effect size for schizophrenia. Overall, although the EE effect is impressive in terms of its predictive power and replicability, these studies are nearly exclusively concerned with symptomatic relapse and, therefore, address a very limited aspect of outcome in schizophrenia. Importantly, there is growing awareness that the range and complexity of outcome in schizophrenia cannot be reflected in the simple relapse dichotomy (Falloon 1988; Lukoff et al. 1984; Strauss and Carpenter 1977).

Additionally, although it may be valuable to assess the degree to which affective attitudes of relatives are expressed, there is a risk that such research promotes the naïve assumption that relatives are solely responsible for the affective climate within the home environment (Strachan et al. 1989). Instead, one can argue that there is a need to examine the reciprocal patterns of influence between patients with schizophrenia and their families. Strachan et al. (1989) appear to be the first group to systematically explore this issue. In their study, they investigated how patients coped with the stressful situation of a discussion with relatives about current problems. Results indicated that parental EE attitudes measured during an inpatient stay strongly predicted patients' transactional behavior after they were discharged. That is, patients interacting with relatives with low EEs made significantly fewer critical and more autonomous statements than those interacting with relatives who had high EEs.

Furthermore, the dominant coping style of the patient was strongly related to the relatives' interactional affective style and EE attitudes. Another study by this same group found that the EE status of a relative evaluated using the CFI was a better predictor of the patient's interactional behavior than of the relative's behavior (Goldstein et al. 1989). Finally, using a different sample of parents and adolescents, Cook et al. (1989) found that mothers with both high and low EEs reciprocated the warmth or coldness shown by their adolescent offspring. Taken together, the results from these investigations support the contention that EE reflects transactional patterns between relatives and patients that are reciprocal and systemic in nature rather than linear and unidirectional (King 1998). At this point, it is impossible to determine who initiates this transactional cycle, but it is clear that reciprocal interactions between patients and relatives are required for its maintenance (Goldstein 1995; King 1998). This approach views the behavior of both patients and relatives as reactions to stress and as attempts to cope with it. In so doing, it implicitly recognizes the role of two moderating variables: the interpretations that each person makes of the other's behavior and the coping skills that each brings to bear (Kavanagh 1992).

In recent years, these issues have begun to be explored in two parallel literatures. Specifically, investigators are now examining the relationship between EE and family burden (Barrowclough and Parle 1997; Jackson et al. 1990; Scazufca and Kuipers 1996, 1998; Smith et al. 1993) and betweeen EE and attributions in relatives of patients with schizophrenia (Barrowclough et al. 1994; Brewin 1988; Brewin et al. 1991; Greenley 1986; Hooley 1985). Only a few studies have systematically investigated the former—that is, the relationship between EE and burden of care. Results indicate that, compared with low-EE relatives, those with high EEs have higher overall levels of objective and subjective burden (Jackson et al. 1990; Scazufca and Kuipers 1996; Smith et al. 1993), perceive themselves as coping less effectively (Barrowclough and Tarrier 1990; Scazufca and Kuipers 1996; Smith et al. 1993), and report higher levels of disturbed behavior in their relatives with schizophrenia (Smith et al. 1993).

Most recently, in an extension of their original work, Scazufca and Kuipers (1998) examined whether changes in EE levels over time were associated with changes in burden of care and relatives' perceptions of patients' social role performance. Patients and relatives were assessed at two points in time: immediately after patient admission, when the patient was in an acute psychotic crisis, and 9 months after discharge from the index admission, when the illness was more stable. Results indicated that for 36% of the relatives, the EE measure was not stable over time; 25% changed from high to low EE, and 11.1% changed from low to high EE. The relatives who changed from high to low EE had greater improvement in feelings of burden and in perceptions of patients' social role performance than the two groups who had stable high or low EE levels (Scazufca and Kuipers 1998). Improvement in relatives' feelings of burden, both objective and subjective, and in perception of patients' social role performance were more accentuated for relatives who changed from high to low EE. Importantly, this occurred despite the fact that there were no objective differences in the severity of psychotic or negative symptoms over time. This finding reinforces the idea that what matters most is the appraisal the relative has of the patient's condition, rather than the actual deficits shown by the patient (Bentsen et al. 1998; Lawton et al. 1989).

In a related, but independent, line of investigation, researchers have begun to explore the relationship between attributions and EE in relatives of patients with schizophrenia (Brewin 1988; Brewin et al. 1991; Greenley 1986; Harrison et al. 1998; Hooley 1985; Weisman et al. 1993, 1998). This work has been driven by the notion that the attributions that families make about the causes of deviant behavior in their ill relative may provide an explanatory framework within which to understand their attitudes toward the patient (i.e., EE) and subsequent coping effectiveness (Harrison and Dadds 1992). This attributional approach draws on a solid theoretical strand within social psychology (Bradbury and Fincham 1987; Lazarus and Folkman 1984) that emphasizes the role of perceived control in coping with stress and illness (Harrison and Dadds 1992).

It is noteworthy that both Hooley (1985) and Greenley (1986) have independently suggested that high EE attitudes reflect attempts to cope by trying to exert control over the perceived consequences of schizophrenia through restoring or changing the patient's behavior. Both investigators have provided modest empirical support for this idea. Additionally, a number of qualitative observations offer indirect support for this contention. For example, Leff and Vaughn (1985) and Jenkins et al. (1987) have noted that low-EE families tend to attribute the cause of the patient's abnormal behavior to a legitimate illness and tended to respect the patient's feelings and perceptions when ill (Weisman et al. 1993). This notion has received further attention by Brewin (1988) and Brewin et al. (1991). Specifically, this group took the indices of EE in 58 relatives of patients with schizophrenia and related them to those relatives' spontaneously expressed causal beliefs about the illness and related symptoms and behaviors. Results suggested that those who were considered high EE because of critical or hostile comments made more attributions to factors internal to, and controllable by, the patient than did relatives who had marked emotional overinvolvement. This latter group was characterized by attributions about the illness that were universal to and uncontrollable by the patient (Brewin et al. 1991). In this respect, emotionally overinvolved relatives were similar to the low EE group.

Weisman et al. (1993, 1998) both replicated and extended these original findings. In their studies, the attributional model of EE was tested first using a sample of 46 Mexican-American families and later with a sample of 40 Anglo-American families of patients with schizophrenia. Consistent with the predictions of this paradigm, they found that high-EE families were more likely than low-EE families to view the illness and associated symptoms as residing within the patient's personal control. Furthermore, those who perceived the patient as having control over the symptoms tended to express greater negative emotions such as anger and annoyance toward the patient than did those who believed the illness was beyond the patient's control. Finally, Barrowclough et al. (1994) used an attributional model of relatives' responses to schizophrenia to explore the relationship between attributions, EE, and patient relapse. This group argued that the EE index should be viewed as an indirect measure of coping responses mediated by beliefs about factors influencing or causing the patient's changed and disturbed behaviors and that high-EE relatives can be distinguished by both the quality and the quantity of their responses to the illness. The results supported their central hypothesis that high-EE relatives made more attributions about illness-related events than did low-EE relatives. Additionally, consistent with the results of earlier studies (Brewin et al. 1991; Weisman et al. 1993), the attributions of overinvolved relatives tended to be more benign than those of other high-EE relatives and were similar to the low-EE group. As predicted, hostile relatives perceived causes as more controllable by and personal to the patient. The most important result that emerged from this investigation was that the attributions made about the illness were more predictive of relapse than the EE status of the relative. That is, rather than the association between relapse and relatives' beliefs being explained by EE, their data suggested the opposite: that any predictive significance of EE was caused by its association with key causal beliefs of the relatives and that these beliefs account for relapse (Barrowclough et al. 1994). A recent extension of this original work has also found some modest support for the notion that appraisal processes underlie parents' reactions to having a relative with schizophrenia and may help both in identifying those at risk of poor adaptation and for developing strategies designed to improve family well-being (Barrowclough and Parle 1997).

Psychoeducational Approaches

In the past 20 years, a considerable literature has developed on psychosocial interventions with families affected by schizophrenia. Not surprisingly, this body of work has been strongly influenced by studies that suggest an association between EE and relapse rates (Vaughn and Leff 1976; Leff and Vaughn 1986). It appears that after clinicians and researchers realized that this construct was consistent with the vulnerability–stress model and accepted that family affective style was linked to the course and outcome of schizophrenia, a move was made to develop programs to alter these interactions (Goldstein and Miklowitz 1995). The assumption was that if negative family attitudes could be modified, relapse rates could be reduced, and if relapse rates were diminished, prognosis would improve.

Reflecting on these interventions, it is clear that psychoeducational approaches (driven by the desire to modify the forces within the home environment that precipitate relapse) have dominated the conceptual landscape. These programs are typically initiated at the point of crisis for the patient and family and may vary in 1) implementation strategies, such as group versus individual approaches; 2) setting, such as home versus clinic; 3) intensity and duration; 4) extent of involvement of the ill relative; 5) credentials and training of providers; and 6) conceptual model (i.e., whether problem-solving skills, communication, or behavioral management are the focus of treatment; Solomon 1996). Taken together, the collective results of this literature offer ample evidence to demonstrate that family treatment oriented toward educating family members and improving their coping skills significantly delays but does not prevent symptomatic relapse (de Jesus Mari and Streiner 1994; Falloon et al. 1982, 1985, 1987; Goldstein et al. 1978; Hogarty et al. 1986, 1991; Lam 1991; Leff et al. 1982, 1985, 1989, 1990; McFarlane 1994; McFarlane et al. 1993, 1995a, 1995b; Randolph et al. 1994; Tarrier et al. 1988, 1989). Specifically, there is considerable evidence indicating that family intervention can reduce relapse rates at 1- and 2-year follow-up (Lam 1991), and recent results suggest that reduced but clinically significant gains can be maintained even at 8-year follow-up (Tarrier et al. 1994). The strongest evidence for the efficacy of these programs comes from trials that have focused on individual family units (Tompson et al. 1996) and, most recently, from multifamily groups (McFarlane et al. 1993, 1995a, 1995b).

Psychoeducational approaches offer several advantages, including a strong conceptual base, efficacy established by increasingly rigorous evaluation, cost effectiveness associated with the reduced need for hospitalization, and the ability to promote collaborative and supportive relationships between families and professionals (Simon et al. 1991). At the same time, however, a number of criticisms have been lodged against these models, many of which are related to the links between the program design and the research methodology (Solomon 1996). For example, the focus of these investigations has been on addressing the question of whether family intervention is effective in reducing relapse rates rather than assessing why these interventions are effective (Budd and Hughes 1997). Consequently, at this time, the mechanisms underlying the efficacy of family interventions and of the various programs relative to one another are still unknown (Bernheim and Lehman 1985; Goldstein 1995; Penn and Mueser 1996; Simon et al. 1991). Despite Lam's (1991) recommendation, no dismantling research design has ever been successfully used to identify which aspects of these interventions explain their effectiveness. Notably, in the absence of data, investigators have speculated that common therapeutic ingredients (i.e., therapeutic alliance, perceived empathy of therapists) or changes in relatives' attributions about the illness account for the efficacy of psychoeducational programs (Barrowclough et al. 1994; Brewin et al. 1991; Budd and Hughes 1997; Harrison and Dadds 1992; Harrison et al. 1998; Weisman et al. 1993, 1998).

In a related vein, several authors (Budd and Hughes 1997; de Jesus Mari and Streiner 1994) have suggested that it is impossible to draw conclusions from this literature that can usefully guide clinical practice because of the nature of the outcome studies that have been conducted to date. Most psychoeducation programs have been designed to fit the requirements of randomized clinical trials, which have had stringent eligibility criteria and thus limited the range of families who participated. Typically, families in these studies were required to have high EE ratings based on the CFI and to have relatively frequent and extensive contact with their relative (Lam 1991; Solomon 1996). Subjects have tended to be white and middle class and to be the parents of the ill relative (Solomon 1996). Given the heterogeneity of families affected by schizophrenia, these findings clearly have limited generalizability (Budd and Hughes 1997; Burland 1998; de Jesus Mari and Streiner 1994; Lam 1991; Solomon

1996), yet they have been applied broadly in clinical practice.

It is noteworthy that these approaches have also achieved only limited acceptance among advocacy groups for families of the mentally ill (Solomon 1996). This lack of acceptance can be attributed to a number of issues, including the concept of EE, which is inextricably linked to psychoeducation and continues to be perceived as blaming families for their relatives' relapses. Emphasis has merely shifted from family factors that cause schizophrenia to those that perpetuate it (Simon et al. 1991; Hatfield 1990, 1994, 1997). Also, treatment is exclusively focused on the behavior of the family even though many other factors may affect the patient and cause relapse (Simon et al. 1991). Finally, despite being referred to as a family intervention, only the well-being of the patient is given real attention (Hatfield et al. 1987; Simon et al. 1991; Solomon 1996), and program effectiveness is measured solely in terms of patient relapse rates.

Family Burden

Currently, one of the biggest criticisms launched against these approaches is that clinicians have been so focused on reducing affectively charged communications that the needs of family caregivers have remained largely overlooked (Hatfield and Lefley 1993; MacCarthy et al. 1989). Work to date has focused largely on how to modify the forces within families that increase the likelihood of symptomatic relapse in patients. Although this may be necessary, clearly the range of disabilities and disruptions of function produced by schizophrenia, as well as the burdens inflicted on families, go far beyond EE and relapse. Too much emphasis has been afforded to the prevention of acute episodes, whereas issues related to family well-being in the face of the complex demands imposed by schizophrenia have not received sufficient attention. This is despite substantial evidence in the literature documenting that the responsibility of providing care for an adult child with schizophrenia can place the caregiver at risk for negative physical, emotional, and social outcomes (Eakes 1995; Oldridge and Hughes 1992; Scottish Schizophrenia Research Group 1992; St-Onge and Lavoie 1997; Winefield and Harvey 1993, 1994).

Compared with studies of family caregiving for relatives with other disabilities and conditions (i.e., Alzheimer's disease, Down syndrome), research investigating the demands of living with a relative with schizophrenia has been slow to develop (Biegel et al. 1991; Hatfield 1997). However, the existing research (Gubman and Tessler 1987; Johnson

1990) has explored the demands of caregiving primarily from the perspective of family burden. Not surprisingly, this work has uncovered significant objective and subjective hardships that include marital problems, disruption of daily routines, social isolation, and financial strain (Creer and Wing 1974; Doll 1976; Gubman and Tessler 1987; Hatfield and Lefley 1993; Johnson 1990; Lefley 1996). Additionally, several investigators have documented considerable distress experienced by families, including grief as a result of feeling as though they have lost a child (MacGregor 1994) or that their child has lost his or her future promise, anxiety about the long-term course of the illness, and sadness related to feeling trapped (Bernheim and Lehman 1985; Lefley 1996; Solomon and Draine 1995; Wasow 1995; Winefield and Harvey 1993, 1994). Although the quality of the available research has varied, no one seems to have seriously questioned the premise that mental illness in a family member can have devastating consequences for the family (Hatfield 1997).

Thus, a corollary to the question of how family intervention affects the course of schizophrenia is: What are the effects of schizophrenia on the family unit (Penn and Mueser 1996)? To some extent, these two questions can be seen as a modern reflection of the dichotomy that still exists in psychiatry between primary and secondary intervention strategies for families (Burland 1998). That is, should education be used as a tool to treat families as toxic agents of relapse in an attempt to prevent illness recurrence or should we work with families to stem the cascade of secondary stressors that threaten their strengths and well-being (Burland 1998)? For the purposes of this discussion, it is suggested that clinicians, researchers, and families will be better served by moving away from existing deficit-based paradigms toward a model of health and illness based on strengths and resources (Walsh 1996). Too often, family distress generated in response to a patient's disturbed, destructive behavior has been labeled as family pathology. Clinicians have erred in confounding family style variance with pathology. For example, the pathologizing label "enmeshed family" has been too readily applied to families that appear to be highly cohesive without acknowledging that the transactional style may be normative for their cultural context or may be a coping strategy that has been adopted to deal with a particular crisis (Walsh 1996). The use of a resiliency-based framework appropriately shifts our attention away from pathology and fault finding and directs us to identify and fortify key interactional processes that enable families to withstand and rebound from the disruptive challenges they face (Walsh 1996). From this vantage point, no single family pattern is regarded as healthy or unhealthy; rather, this approach sees a broad range of family forms as normative and moves us in the direction of examining the goodness of fit between a family's style, with its particular strengths and vulnerabilities, and the biopsychosocial demands of the illness over time (Rolland 1994).

Creating a Framework for Intervention with Families Dealing with a First Episode of Psychosis

Interventions in psychosis, whether biological or psychosocial, have generally ignored the phase and age of onset of the illness (Birchwood et al. 1998). Consequently, one of the primary difficulties at this juncture is the lack of a coherent framework that considers the unfolding of illness-related developmental tasks after the onset of the illness. But without this theoretical blueprint, it becomes difficult to explore meaningful clinical strategies for work with first-episode families. It is suggested, therefore, that the time has come to ask a different question: what information and support should be provided for families during the different phases of schizophrenia that will make a difference in their ability to cope and adapt (Rolland 1994)?

A framework for exploring the illness trajectory with the common issues and challenges faced by families is presented below and provides a conceptual base for approaching clinical practice and research regarding the impact of schizophrenia from a family systems perspective. This framework represents a synthesis of the work of Rolland (1994) and McGorry (1992) and the personal narratives of affected families. Three major phases are described: 1) the prodrome and the first crisis, 2) the initial period of adjustment, and 2) the development of a long-term illness. It is suggested that each phase has its own unique demands and developmental tasks that may require significantly different strengths, attitudes, or changes from families (Rolland 1994).

Prodrome and First Crisis

Nothing can prepare families for the shock and devastation of watching a child become totally consumed and incapacitated by psychosis. It is frightening and overwhelming, ransacks lives with an unimaginable ferocity, and reverberates throughout families leaving no one untouched. When psychosis first strikes, families are usually unaware of the nature and magnitude of the problem. Through no fault of their own, subtle changes in behavior are often attributed to other causes, most often adolescence. It is only after the disruptive or disturbed behavior persists that families come to realize that the family member's problem is not going to disappear spontaneously and that he or she may even need professional attention. Families typically begin an extensive search for an explanation and help.

Eventually, there is some recognition that the difficulties may be psychiatric. As this reality starts to sink in, families are faced with the formidable challenge of having to come to grips with the possibility that their child has a serious mental illness. Regardless of whether the illness developed acutely or insidiously, its novelty means that the experience is highly threatening and easily misunderstood by families (McGorry 1992). At this time, families have a strong need for reassurance that they are handling things normally. Admission to a hospital or an outpatient program brings with it a whole host of reactions. The fear and anxiety are palpable. Parents have retrospectively reported that during this initial crisis they were confused and dazed and, at times, felt as though they were in a trance and unable to comprehend what was happening. To make matters worse, they were asked to hand over the care of their child to strangers. Although at one level this temporary relinquishing of responsibility can provide a sense of relief, the experience also provokes anxiety. It is as if the admission into care confirms their worst fears—that something is terribly wrong with their child. There are new faces, new rules, and new routines to learn, and of course a multitude of questions that get played over and over again: What is happening to my child? How did this happen? Why him/her? Why us? Will this ever go away? Is this schizophrenia? Will life ever be the same?

Initial Period of Adjustment

Discussions with health care providers about the nature of the illness and its prognosis and about prescriptions for management constitute a framing event for families (Rolland 1994). This is a period of excruciating vulnerability and uncertainty in which families search for ways to reestablish the control in their lives that has been taken away by the illness. The inability to protect their child from illness and suffering can, at times, be an overwhelming assault on their parental identity as protectors and providers. There is an oppressive sense of failure and a deep sense of being violated. Additionally, the anticipation of loss becomes an overarching issue for most. Even after the psychosis is under control, the "deskilling" (i.e., problems with memory, concentration, organization, and motivation; depression; changes in personality) that usually accompanies a first episode of psychosis serves as a constant reminder that the future is uncertain and potentially fraught with more serious and persistent problems. Anticipatory loss generates a range of intensified emotional and interactional responses among families, including anxiety, anger, existential aloneness, denial, sadness, disappointment, resentment, guilt, exhaustion, and desperation. There may be intense ambivalence toward the ill family member with vacillations between wishes for closeness and fantasies of escape from an unbearable situation (Rolland 1994). There is also a risk of becoming hypervigilant and overprotective.

During the first two phases, there are several key adaptive tasks for families. These include learning about the illness and its course and treatment; creating a meaning for the illness that maximizes the preservation of mastery and competence for family members in a context of partial loss and possible further deterioration; learning to deal with symptoms; adapting to the hospital or clinic environments and to treatment procedures associated with schizophrenia; and establishing and maintaining positive relationships with the health care team (McGorry 1992; Rolland 1994). Because serious illness in a loved one is often experienced as a fundamental betrayal (Kleinman 1988), the creation of an empowering narrative is a formidable task for many (Rolland 1994). Clinicians can help families overcome feelings of helplessness and vulnerability by involving them from the outset. Families need to believe that they have allies in their personal battle against schizophrenia. They need to know that their observations and perceptions are valued and integrated into treatment planning; they need education about the illness that is paced in a manageable way; and they need a chance to be heard and to relate their own account of their child's illness, his or her life, and the life of the family (Rolland 1994). All of these approaches go a long way toward establishing a working relationship between families and health care providers that is based on trust and mutual respect. This in turn increases the likelihood that anxiety about an uncertain future will be managed in a way that enables families to not lose sight of the possibilities of recovery and rehabilitation.

Development of a Long-Term Illness

The question of permanency lurks in the minds of all families after the onset of a first episode of psychosis—that is, will their child ever completely recover and be well again? Unfortunately, the answer to this question is usually available only after many months, and sometimes years, of uncertainty and ambiguity. In acute health crises that are resolved within days, weeks, or months, a focus on good biomedical care takes priority.

Psychosocial demands on families may be intense, but they are time limited (Rolland 1994). However, for many patients, the first episode is not simply a short-term crisis that will resolve and go away. Rather, it is the beginning of an episodic illness that will fluctuate for years between periods of acute exacerbations of symptoms and periods of improvement or stability (Wing 1986).

There is little doubt that after this threshold is crossed there are further painful and disorganizing consequences for families (Hatfield and Lefley 1993; Hatfield et al. 1987). There is consensus that an extreme sense of loss can be expected among parents who learn that their child has developed a more disabling form of schizophrenia (Sargent and Liebman 1985). This is based on the recognition that, for parents, the disability represents the loss of the wished-for "normal child" and of the known, previously nondisabled person (Hillyer-Davis 1987). A child is both a biological and psychological extension of his or her parents (Rando 1986). Thus, when a child develops a severe and persistent mental illness such as schizophrenia, parents have already accumulated an array of past images and experiences. These form the basis on which they project future hopes for the child (Terkelsen 1987). After a more long-term illness declares itself, existing hopes, dreams, and expectations for the child, the family, and the future need to be mourned and power, roles, and responsibilities need to be reassigned (Hatfield et al. 1987).

Several studies (Atkinson 1994; Davis and Schultz 1998; Miller 1996; Miller et al. 1990; Solomon and Draine 1995) are now available that provide convincing evidence that families of the mentally ill experience measurable and sustained grief comparable in magnitude with that of those who have experienced a death. However, the grief associated with long-term mental illness is perhaps, in some ways, more difficult and enduring. The lack of finality, for example, can hinder acceptance and allow parents to cling to the hope that the illness and associated disability will spontaneously remit. Additionally, not only does the child with schizophrenia not die, but he or she also requires more care than do other children (Hillyer-Davis 1987). Consequently, to resolve grief in the traditional sense would require denial of the continuity of the child's life. Because children with schizophrenia remain both physically and psychologically present, it seems more helpful to consider family responses as natural reactions to an ongoing, often tragic experience, one that is not time bound (Hillyer-Davis 1987). Ideally, parents must master their grief concerning both their child and those aspects of family life that are lost to the illness.

In addition to having to contend with prolonged and sustained grief, families are faced with caregiving demands that often give rise to exhaustion and ambivalence as financial and emotional resources become depleted (Rolland 1994). There are two important and related questions that arise for families at this time. First, how do they balance their obligations to their ill family member with their own needs? Second, how do they maintain a semblance of a normal life under the abnormal conditions imposed by chronic schizophrenia (Rolland 1994)?

Conclusions and Recommendations

In the past 20–25 years, a shift has occurred in the conceptualization of the role of social and family factors in schizophrenia (Barrowclough and Tarrier 1984). In place of causal relationships, investigators have moved to explore aspects of the home environment that sustain the illness after it has appeared. The research from the United Kingdom on EE has been influential in solidifying this paradigm shift within psychiatry and has been the driving force behind the psychoeducation movement. Importantly, during the past two decades tremendous progress has been made in providing information to families affected by schizophrenia and involving them as partners in the rehabilitation process. At the same time, however, the range of helping responses available has narrowed. Psychoeducation has become an overgeneralized approach because insufficient stock has been taken of the complexity of caregiving over time.

Thus, it is suggested that we reframe our thinking about families affected by schizophrenia in ways that will allow us to move beyond existing limitations (Cook et al. 1997). Research and clinical experience repeatedly remind us that schizophrenia often wreaks havoc with an unimaginable ferocity. It is suggested, therefore, that the time has come to systematically address two broad but related questions. First, what contributes to family well-being after the advent of schizophrenia? And second, how do we prepare families to cope in ways that preserve their strengths? One fundamental assumption embedded in this work is that clinical care and effective coping and adaptation can best occur within an environment that is family centered, contextual, and collaborative (Rolland 1994) and that above all begins during the first episode.

Living well with the stresses and uncertainties of schizophrenia can be a monumental challenge (Rolland 1994). Although each family's experience of schizophrenia is unique and cannot be reduced to a simple clinical formula, there are predictable issues that can help guide a family's quest for meaning and mastery of the challenges (Rolland 1994). A beginning framework has been offered that attempts to delineate some of the core practical and emotional demands faced by families after the onset of a family member's schizophrenia. At the most general level, the utility of this approach must be evaluated. After the relevance of this approach has been demonstrated, exciting and bountiful vistas will emerge for research into family intervention designed to optimize outcome after the onset of schizophrenia.

The following quotation, written by the mother of a young man who received treatment in our program, eloquently summarizes the range and intensity of emotions that parents often experience:

> A long time before our son became ill, we knew that he was "different." The so-called phases we thought he was going through—his shyness, loneliness, withdrawal, and inability to concentrate and to make decisions; his speaking to himself; his preoccupation with mystical things, UFOs, flights into wild fantasies, hell, the devil, and more—were taking away his sense of reality, his common sense. We knew that he wouldn't have it easy in his life, but we didn't realize that he was already walking on the edge and that his thin red line was already breaking.
>
> Eventually that day came, that terrible, never-to-be-forgotten day, when, looking into his eyes, I witnessed his transition from sanity into insanity. And I knew…we knew.
>
> The first feelings were FEAR and PAIN. A terrible fear, a mortal fear, as if someone had pushed me into an abyss. It awoke in me an instinct for protection. I felt like a beast whose newborn was in danger. I wanted to grab my son and run out of harm's way to some hidden corner of the world. Fear of the known and unknown: What is going to happen to him? Who is going to take care of him if something happens to us? In my mind's eye, I saw him wandering aimlessly around, alone, lost, neglected, forgotten, ridiculed. The terrible images of psychiatric patients from *One Flew Over the Cuckoo's Nest, Suddenly Lost in Summer, Snake Pit*, and many more magnified that fear.
>
> Feeling of sadness. Profound, as if I have lost him, a presence of death. Dread, dread that wakes you in the middle of the night, blind desperation. Tears. I cried all the time, everywhere: on the streets, at work, at church. I found myself literally choking in tears.
>
> And the GUILT. That most useless and destructive feeling of all. Where did we go wrong? Who did what? So many ifs. If only we didn't push him to study, didn't lecture him, didn't insist on order!
>
> Denial. Maybe the doctor is wrong. Let's not tell anybody; maybe he will pull himself together, snap out of it.
>
> Mistrust. How come this medication doesn't work? We should change the doctor.
>
> How did I deal with these feelings, dilemmas, this roller coaster of emotions I found myself on?

The instinct for protection led me to take my son on a trip, on several trips, but his delusions didn't stop at the borders. I started to look around, as if I was scanning with his eyes the potential danger and threat. I have slowly been drawn into his underworld. I started to read excessively everything available about schizophrenia, underlining all the now familiar signs and symptoms, and I was devastated.

My son said, "I am losing control over my mind; something is happening to me." "I feel nothing, empty." Or "I feel pain in my soul, in my heart."

His is a grave illness. In what other disease does the patient not understand, cannot grasp what is going on, cannot say: "I am going to fight this and I am going to win"? His pain cannot be measured on a scale from 1 to 10. In his world, the logic is lost; the definitions lose their meaning and objectivity is replaced with deluded ideas; things develop another dimension.

I did two things at first: found myself a doctor who let me unburden my troubles and I started to attend meetings for parents or spouses—a support group. That helped me a little, but I think I was doing too many things at the same time.

My real break came when our son was admitted to hospital. It didn't mean that I suffered less or that our son was cured. It meant that I had found a group of people who were trying their utmost to help my son. Here I have found understanding, compassion, patience, and information, but most of all, here I have been included, as a parent, in planning my son's care and for his well being. Thanks to the staff, I don't feel alone, don't feel guilty, and I have HOPE.

My strength also comes from my faith. In the beginning, I tried to bargain with God. I said, "If you take this illness from my son, I'll do anything. Take everything from me. Take my life." Or I would turn to him reproachingly: "What are you punishing us for?" But that's not what faith is all about! It is, rather, about purpose, love, acceptance, spirituality, and hope—and today, my strength is nurtured on those.

The other source of strength came from maintaining the unity and traditions within my family. "Take each day as it comes" is no longer an empty phrase.

The world that I used to call unjustly "an underworld," the world of shadowy figures I passed by on the streets, that world I always managed to push into the periphery of my mind. Today, the shadowy figures have become real people; they are the ones I want to love and embrace. Nothing is as it was before.

People tell me, "You have to have a life of your own!" I don't know what they mean. This is my life, and my son is the most important part of it. My happiness is measured by his well-being. When I step into the fine spring morning and thank God for its beauty, I feel that in this vast universe there must be a reason for everything.

We have to break the walls of silence, whispers, shame, guilt, ignorance, and misconceptions about mental illness. We must be the eyes, ears, and, often, the minds of our children. We must knock on doors, ask for more help so that research can go on. We mustn't let our children go gently into that Good Night. Most of all, we must give them our unconditional love. Only then can we say that we have truly done our best, that we have truly become our brother's keepers.

Ana, 1994

References

Atkinson SD: Grieving and loss in parents with a schizophrenic child. Am J Psychiatry 151:1137–1139, 1994

Barrelet L, Ferrero F, Szigethy L, et al: Expressed emotion and first admission schizophrenia. Br J Psychiatry 156:357–362, 1990

Barrowclough C, Parle M: Appraisal, psychological adjustment and expressed emotion in relatives of patients suffering from schizophrenia. Br J Psychiatry 171:26–30, 1997

Barrowclough C, Tarrier N: Psychosocial interventions with families and their effects on the course of schizophrenia: a review. Psychol Med 14:629–642, 1984

Barrowclough C, Tarrier N: Social functioning in schizophrenic patients, I: the effects of expressed emotion and family intervention. Soc Psychiatry Psychiatr Epidemiol 25:125–130, 1990

Barrowclough C, Johnson M, Tarrier N: Attributions, expressed emotion and patient relapse: an attributional model of relatives' responses to schizophrenic illness. Behav Ther 25:67–88, 1994

Bateson G, Jackson D, Haley J, et al: Toward a theory of schizophrenia. Behav Sci 1:251–264, 1956

Bellack A, Mueser K: Psychosocial treatment for schizophrenia. Schizophr Bull 19:317–336, 1993

Bentsen H, Notland TH, Boye B, et al: Criticism and hostility in relatives of patients with schizophrenia or related psychosis: demographic and clinical predictors. Acta Psychiatr Scand 97:76–85, 1998

Bernheim K, Lehman AF: Working with Families of the Mentally Ill. New York, WW Norton, 1985

Biegel DE, Sales E, Schulz R: Family caregiving in chronic illness. Newbury Park, CA, Sage, 1991

Birchwood M, MacMillan F: Early intervention in schizophrenia. Aust NZ J Psychiatry 27:374–378, 1993

Birchwood M, Todd P, Jackson C: Early intervention in psychosis: the critical period hypothesis. Br J Psychiatry 172(suppl 33):53–59, 1998

Black D, Andreasen N: Schizophrenia, schizophreniform disorder and delusional (paranoid) disorder, in The American Psychiatric Press Textbook of Psychiatry, 2nd Edition. Edited by Hales R, Yudofsky S, Talbot J. Washington, DC, American Psychiatric Press, 1994, pp 411–464

Bradbury TN, Fincham FD: Affect and cognition in close relationships: towards an integrative model. Cognition and Emotion 1:59–87, 1987

Breier A, Screiber J, Dyer J, et al: National Institute of Mental Health longitudinal study of chronic schizophrenia. Arch Gen Psychiatry 48:239–246, 1991

Brewin CR: Cognitive Foundations of Clinical Psychology. London, England, Erlbaum, 1988

Brewin CR, MacCarthy B, Duda K, et al: Attributions and expressed emotion in the relatives of patients with schizophrenia. J Abnorm Psychol 100:546–554, 1991

Brown G: Experiences of discharged chronic schizophrenic mental hospital patients in various types of living groups. Millbank Memorial Fund Quarterly 37:105–131, 1959

Brown G, Rutter M: The measurement of family activities and relationships: a methodological study. Human Relations 19:241–263, 1966

Brown G, Carstairs GM, Topping GC: The post hospital adjustment of chronic mental patients. Lancet II:685–689, 1958

Brown G, Monck E, Carstairs G, et al: Influence of family life on the course of schizophrenic illness. British Journal of Preventative Social Medicine 36:55–68, 1962

Brown G, Birley J, Wing J: Influence of family life on the course of schizophrenic disorders: a replication. Br J Psychiatry 121:241–258, 1972

Budd R, Hughes I: What do relatives of people with schizophrenia find helpful about family intervention? Schizophr Bull 23:341–346, 1997

Burland J: Family to family: a trauma and recovery model of family education. New Dir Ment Health Serv 77:33–69, 1998

Butzlaff R, Hooley J: Expressed emotion and psychiatric relapse: a metaanalysis. Arch Gen Psychiatry 55:547–552, 1998

Ciompi L: Learning from outcome studies: toward a comprehensive biological-psychosocial understanding of schizophrenia. Schizophr Res 1:373–384, 1988

Cook WL, Strachan AM, Goldstein MJ, et al: Expressed emotion and reciprocal affective relationships in the families of disturbed adolescents. Family Process 28:337–348, 1989

Cook J, Pickett S, Coehler C: Families of adults with severe mental illness: the next generation of research. Introduction. Am J Orthopsychiatry 67:172–176, 1997

Creer C, Wing J: Schizophrenia At Home. London, England, National Schizophrenia Fellowship, 1974

Davis D, Schultz C: Grief, parenting and schizophrenia. Soc Sci Med 46:369–379, 1998 de Jesus Mari J, Streiner D: An overview of family interventions and relapse on schizophrenia: meta-analysis of research findings. Psychol Med 24, 565–578, 1994

Doll W: Family coping with the mentally ill: an unanticipated problem of deinstitutionalization, in Mental Disorder in Social Context. Edited by Greenley JR. Greenwich, CT, JAI Press, 1976, pp 203–236

Dulz B, Hand I: Short term relapse in young schizophrenics: can it be predicted and affected by family (CFI), patient and treatment variables, in Treatment of Schizophrenia. Edited by Goldstein M, Hand I, Hawlweg K. Berlin, Germany, Springer-Verlag, 1986, pp 59–85

Eakes G: Chronic sorrow: the lived experience of parents of chronically mentally ill. Arch Psychiatr Nurs 9:77–84, 1995

Falloon I: Expressed emotion: current status. Psychol Med 18:269–274, 1988

Falloon I, Boyd J, McGill C: Family management in the prevention of exacerbations of schizophrenia: a controlled study. N Engl J Med 300:1437–1440, 1982

Falloon I, Boyd J, McGill C: Family care of schizophrenia: a problem solving approach to the treatment of mental illness. New York, Guilford Press, 1984

Falloon I, Boyd J, Williamson M, et al: Family management in the prevention of morbidity of schizophrenia: clinical outcome of a two-year longitudinal study. Arch Gen Psychiatry 42:887–986, 1985

Falloon I, McGill C, Boyd J, et al: Family management in the prevention of morbidity of schizophrenia: social outcome of a two year longitudinal study. Psychol Med 17:59–66, 1987

Falloon I, Hahlweg K, Tarrier N: Family intervention in the community management of schizophrenia, in Schizophrenia: Concepts, Vulnerability, and Interventions. Edited by Straube ER, Hahlweg K. New York, Springer-Verlag, 1990, pp 217–240

Freeman H: Relationship of schizophrenia to the environment. Br J Psychiatry 155(suppl 5):90–99, 1989

Fromm-Reichmann F: Notes on the development of treatment of schizophrenia by psychoanalytic psychotherapy. Psychiatry 11:263–273, 1948

Glynn S, Randolph E, Eth S, et al. Patient psychopathology and expressed emotion in schizophrenia. Br J Psychiatry 157:877–880, 1990

Goldstein M: Transactional processes associated with relatives' expressed emotion. Int J Ment Health 24:76–96, 1995

Goldstein M, Miklowitz D: The effectiveness of psychoeducational family therapy in the treatment of schizophrenic disorders. J Marital Fam Ther 21:361–376, 1995

Goldstein M, Rodnick E, Evans J: Drug and family therapy in the aftercare of acute schizophrenics. Arch Gen Psychiatry 35:1169–1177, 1978

Goldstein M, Miklowitz DJ, Strachan AS, et al: Patterns of expressed emotion and patient coping styles that characterize the families of recent onset schizophrenics. Br J Psychiatry 155(suppl 5):107–111, 1989

Greenley JR: Social control and expressed emotion. J Nerv Ment Dis 174:24–30, 1986

Gubman G, Tessler R: The impact of mental illness on families. Journal of Family Issues 8:226–245, 1987

Harrison C, Dadds M: Attributions of symptomatology: an exploration of family factors associated with expressed emotion. Aust NZ J Psychiatry 26:408–416, 1992

Harrison C, Dadds M, Smith G: Family caregivers' criticism of patients with schizophrenia. Psychiatr Serv 49:918–924, 1998

Hatfield A: Family education in mental illness, in Families of the Mentally Ill: Coping and Adaptation. Edited by Hatfield A, Lefley H. New York, Guilford, 1990

Hatfield A: Developing collaborative relationships with families. New Dir Ment Health Serv 62:51–59, 1994

Hatfield A: Families of adults with severe mental illness: new directions in research. Am J Orthopsychiatry 67:254–260, 1997

Hatfield A, Lefley H: Surviving Mental Illness: Stress, Coping and Adaptation. New York, Guilford, 1993

Hatfield A, Spaniol L, Zipple AM: Expressed emotion: a family perspective Schizophr Bull 13:221–226, 1987

Hillyer-Davis B: Disability and grief. Social Casework: Journal of Contemporary Social Work 68:352–357, 1987

Hogarty G: Expressed emotion and schizophrenic relapse: implications from the Pittsburgh study, in Controversies in Schizophrenia. Edited by Alpert M. New York, Guilford, 1985, pp 354–365

Hogarty G, Anderson C, Reiss D: Family psychoeducation, social skills training, and maintenance chemotherapy in the aftercare treatment of schizophrenia, I: one-year effects of a controlled study on relapse and expressed emotion. Arch Gen Psychiatry 43:633–642, 1986

Hogarty G, McEvoy J, Munetz M, et al: Dose fluphenazine, familial expressed emotion and outcome in schizophrenia: results of a 2-year controlled study. Arch Gen Psychiatry 45:797–805, 1988

Hogarty G, Anderson C, Reiss D, et al: Family psychoeducation, social skills training, and maintenance chemotherapy in the aftercare treatment of schizophrenia. Arch Gen Psychiatry 48:340–347, 1991

Hooley JM: Expressed emotion: a review of the critical literature. Clin Psychol Rev 5:119–139, 1985

Jackson HJ, Smith N, McGorry P: Relationship between expressed emotion and family burden in psychotic disorders: an exploratory study. Acta Psychiatr Scand 82:243–249, 1990

Jenkins JH, Karno M, de la Selva A, et al: Expressed emotion in cross cultural context: familial responses to schizophrenic illness among Mexican Americans, in Treatment of Schizophrenia: Family Assessment and Intervention. Edited by Goldstein MJ, Hand I, Hahlweg K. New York, Springer-Verlag, 1987, pp 35–49

Johnson D: The expectation of outcome from maintenance therapy in chronic schizophrenic patients. Br J Psychiatry 128:246–250, 1976

Johnson D: The family's experience of living with mental illness, in Families as Allies in the Treatment of the Mentally Ill: New Directions for Mental Health Professionals. Edited by Lefley H, Johnson D. Washington, DC, American Psychiatric Press, 1990, pp 31–63

Kavanagh DJ: Recent developments in expressed emotion and schizophrenia. Br J Psychiatry 160:601–620, 1992

Kay S: Significance of positive-negative distinction in schizophrenia. Schizophr Bull 16:635–652, 1990

King S: Is expressed emotion cause or effect? A longitudinal study. Int Clin Psychopharmacol 13(suppl 1):107–108, 1998

Kleinman A: The Illness Narratives: Suffering, Healing, and the Human Condition. New York, Basic Books, 1988

Kuipers L: The measurement of expressed emotion: its influence on research and clinical practice. Int Rev Psychiatry 6:187–199, 1994

Lam D: Psychosocial family intervention in schizophrenia: a review of empirical studies. Psychol Med 21:423–441, 1991

Lawton MP, Kleban MH, Moss M, et al: Measuring caregiving appraisal. J Gerontol 44:61–71, 1989

Lazarus R, Folkman S: Coping and adaptation, in The Handbook of Behavioral Medicine. Edited by Gentry D. New York, Guilford, 1984, pp 282–325

Leff J, Vaughn C: Expressed Emotion in Families. New York, Guilford, 1985

Leff J, Vaughn C: First episodes of schizophrenia. Br J Psychiatry 148:215–216, 1986

Leff J, Wing J: Trial of maintenance therapy in schizophrenia. BMJ 3:599–604, 1971

Leff J, Kuipers L, Berkowitz R, et al: A controlled trial of intervention in families of schizophrenic patients. Br J Psychiatry 141:121–134, 1982

Leff J, Kuipers L, Berkowitz R, et al: A controlled trial of social intervention in the families of schizophrenic patients: two-year follow up. Br J Psychiatry 146:594–600, 1985

Leff J, Berkowitz R, Shavit N, et al: A trial of family therapy versus a relatives' group for schizophrenia. Br J Psychiatry 154:58–66, 1989

Leff J, Berkowitz R, Shavit N, et al: A trial of family therapy versus a relatives' group for schizophrenia: two year followup. Br J Psychiatry 157:571–577, 1990

Lefley H: Family Caregiving and Mental Illness. Thousand Oaks, CA, Sage, 1996

Lukoff D, Snyder K, Ventura J, et al: Life events, familial stress and coping in the developmental course of schizophrenia. Schizophr Bull 10:258–292, 1984

MacCarthy B, Kuipers L, Hurry J, et al: Counseling the relatives of the long-term adult mentally ill, I: evaluation of the impact on relatives and patients. Br J Psychiatry 154:768–775, 1989

MacGregor P: Grief: the unrecognized parental response to mental illness in a child. Social Work 39:160–166, 1994

MacMillan JF, Gold A, Crow TJ, et al: Expressed emotion and relapse in schizophrenia. Br J Psychiatry 148:741–744, 1986a

MacMillan JF, Gold A, Crow TJ, et al: The Northwick Park study of first episode schizophrenia, IV: expressed emotion and relapse. Br J Psychiatry 148:133–143, 1986b

McFarlane WR: Multiple family groups and psychoeducation in the treatment of schizophrenia. New Dir Ment Health Serv 62:13–22, 1994

McFarlane WR, Dunne E, Lukens E, et al: From research to clinical practice: dissemination of New York State's family psychoeducational project. Hospital and Community Psychiatry 44:265–270, 1993

McFarlane WR, Lukens E, Link B, et al: The multiple family group, psychoeducation and maintenance medication in the treatment of schizophrenia. Arch Gen Psychiatry 52:679–687, 1995a

McFarlane WR, Link B, Dushay R, et al: Psychoeducational multiple family groups: four-year relapse outcome in schizophrenia. Family Process 34:127–144, 1995b

McGlashan T: Psychosocial treatments, in Schizophrenia: From Mind to Molecule. Edited by Andreasen N. Washington, DC, American Psychiatric Press, 1994, pp 189–214

McGlashan T: Early detection and intervention of schizophrenia: rationale and research. Br J Psychiatry 172(suppl):3–6, 1998

McGorry P: The concept of recovery and secondary prevention in psychotic disorders. Aust NZ J Psychiatry 26:3–17, 1992

Miller F: Grief therapy for relatives of persons with serious mental illness. Psychiatr Serv 47:633–637, 1996

Miller F, Dworkin J, Ward M, et al: A preliminary study of unresolved grief in families of seriously mentally ill patients. Hospital and Community Psychiatry 41:1321–1325, 1990

Nuechterlein K, Dawson M: A heuristic vulnerability-stress model of schizophrenic episodes. Schizophr Bull 10:300–312, 1984

Nuechterlein K, Dawson M, Gitlin G, et al: Developmental processes in schizophrenia disorders: longitudinal studies of vulnerability and stress. Schizophr Bull 18:387–425, 1992

Oldridge ML, Hughes ICT: Psychological well being in families with a member suffering from schizophrenia: an investigation into longstanding problems. Br J Psychiatry 161:249–251, 1992

Parker G, Johnson P, Hayward L: Parental expressed emotion as a predictor of schizophrenia relapse. Arch Gen Psychiatry 45:806–813, 1988

Penn D, Mueser K: Research update on the psychosocial treatment of schizophrenia. Am J Psychiatry 153:607–617, 1996

Rando T: Parental Loss of a Child. Champagne, IL, Research Press, 1986

Randolph ET, Eth S, Glynn SM, et al: Behavioral family management in schizophrenia: outcome of a clinical-based inventory. Br J Psychiatry 164:501–506, 1994

Rolland J: Families, Illness and Disability. New York, Basic Books, 1994

Rutter M: Psychosocial resilience and protective mechanisms. Am J Orthopsychiatry 57:316–331, 1987

Sargent J, Liebman R: Childhood chronic illness: issues for psychotherapists. Community Ment Health J 21:294–311, 1985

Scazufca M, Kuipers L: Links between expressed emotion and burden of care in relatives of patients with schizophrenia. Br J Psychiatry 168:580–587, 1996

Scazufca M, Kuipers L: Stability of expressed emotion in relatives of those with schizophrenia and its relationship with burden of care and perception of patients' social functioning. Psychol Med 28:453–461, 1998

Scottish Schizophrenia Research Group: The Scottish First Episode Schizophrenia Study, VIII: five year follow up: clinical and psychosocial findings. Br J Psychiatry 161:496–500, 1992

Simon C, McNeil J, Franklin C, et al: The family and schizophrenia: toward a psychoeducational approach. Families in Society: The Journal of Contemporary Human Services 13:323–331, 1991

Smith J, Birchwood M, Cochrane R, et al: The needs of high and low expressed emotion families: a normative approach. Soc Psychiatry Psychiatr Epidemiol 28:11–16, 1993

Solomon P: Moving from psychoeducation to family education for families of adults with serious mental illness. Psychiatr Serv 47:1364–1370, 1996

Solomon P: The cultural context of interventions for family members with a seriously mentally ill relative. New Dir Ment Health Serv 77:5–16, 1998

Solomon P, Draine J: Subjective burden among family members of mentally ill adults: relationship to stress, coping and adaptation. Am J Orthopsychiatry 65:419–426, 1995

Stirling J, Tantam D, Thomas P, et al: Expressed emotion and early onset schizophrenia: the ontogeny of EE during an 18 month follow up. Psychol Med 23:771–778, 1993

Strachan AM, Leff JP, Goldstein MJ, et al: Emotional attitudes and direct communication in the families of schizophrenics: a cross national replication. Br J Psychiatry 149:279–287, 1986

Strachan AM, Feingold D, Goldstein MJ, et al: Is expressed emotion an index of a transactional process? II: patient's coping style. Family Process 28:169–181, 1989

Strauss J, Carpenter WT: Prediction of outcome in schizophrenia, III: five-year outcome and its predictors. Arch Gen Psychiatry 34:159–163, 1977

Strauss J, Hafez H, Lieberman P, et al: The course of psychiatric disorders, III: longitudinal principles. Am J Psychiatry 142:289–296, 1985

St-Onge M, Lavoie F: The experience of caregiving among mothers of adults suffering from psychotic disorders: factors associated with their psychological distress. Am J Community Psychol 25:73–94, 1997

Syvalanti EK: Biological factors in schizophrenia: structure and functional aspects. Br J Psychiatry 158(suppl 23):9–14, 1994

Szmukler GI, Eisler I, Russell GFM, et al: Anorexia nervosa, parental expressed emotion and dropping out of treatment. Br J Psychiatry 147:265–271, 1985

Szmukler GI, Berkowitz R, Eisler I, et al: Expressed emotion in individual and family settings: a comparative study. Br J Psychiatry 151:174–178, 1987

Tarrier N, Barrowclough C, Vaughn C, et al: The community management of schizophrenia: a controlled trial of a behavioral intervention with families to reduce relapse. Br J Psychiatry 153:532–542, 1988

Tarrier N, Barrowclough C, Vaughn C, et al: The community management of schizophrenia: a two-year follow-up of a behavioral intervention with families. Br J Psychiatry 154:625–628, 1989

Tarrier N, Barrowclough C, Porceddu K, et al: The Salford Family Intervention Project: relapse rates of schizophrenia at 5 and 8 years. Br J Psychiatry 165:829–832, 1994

Terkelsen K: The evolution of family responses to mental illness through time, in Families of the Mentally Ill: Coping and Adaptation. Edited by Hatfield A, Lefley H. New York, Guilford, 1987, pp 151–166

Tompson M, Goldstein M, Rea M: Psychoeducational family intervention: individual differences in response to treatment, in Advanced Prelapse Education Compliance and Relapse in Practice. Edited by Kane J, van den Bosch RJ. Amsterdam, The Netherlands, Lundbeck Symposium, 1996, pp 21–28

Vaughn C, Leff J: The influence of family and social factors on the course of psychiatric illness: a comparison of schizophrenia and depressed neurotic patients. Br J Psychiatry 129:125–137, 1976

Vaughn C, Snyder K, Jones S, et al: Family factors in schizophrenic relapse: replication in California of British research on expressed emotion. Arch Gen Psychiatry 41:1169–1177, 1984

Vaughn C, Doyle M, McConaghy N, et al: The Sydney intervention trial: a controlled trial of relatives' counseling to reduce schizophrenic relapse. Soc Psychiatry Psychiatr Epidemiol 27:16–21, 1992

Walsh F: Families and mental illness: What have we learned? in Mental Illness in the Family: Issues and Trends. Edited by Abosh B, Collins A. Toronto, Canada, University of Toronto Press, 1996, pp 26–37

Wasow M: Chronic schizophrenia and Alzheimer's disease: the losses for parents, spouses and children compared. J Chron Dis 38:711–716, 1995

Weisman, A, Lopez SR, Regeser-Karno M, et al: An attributional analysis of expressed emotion in Mexican American families with schizophrenia. J Abnorm Psychol 102:601–606, 1993

Weisman A, Nuechterlein K, Goldstein M, et al: Expressed emotion, attributions and schizophrenia symptoms dimensions. J Abnorm Psychol 107:355–359, 1998

Wing J: Chronic schizophrenia and long term hospitalization. Br J Psychiatry 152:144–145, 1986

Winefield H, Harvey E: Determinants of psychological distress in relatives of people with chronic schizophrenia. Schizophr Bull 19:619–626, 1993

Winefield H, Harvey E: Needs of family caregivers in chronic schizophrenia. Schizophr Bull 20:557–566, 1994

Zisook S: Biopsychosocial Aspects of Bereavement. Washington, DC, American Psychiatric Press, 1987

Zubin J, Spring B: Vulnerability: a new view of schizophrenia. J Abnorm Psychol 86:103–126, 1977

PART III

Neurobiological Investigations of the Early Stages of Schizophrenia

7

Childhood-Onset Schizophrenia

Research Update

Sanjiv Kumra, M.D.

Robert Nicolson, M.D.

Judith L. Rapoport, M.D.

Schizophrenia can be conceptualized as a complex biological disorder in which genes play a role and in which brain development is likely to be abnormal (Barondes et al. 1997). Although twin, family, and adoption studies suggest that genetic factors are of substantial etiologic importance, these may not be present in all instances, pointing to the participation of other factors (Gershon et al. 1998). The fact that most cases of schizophrenia arise in early adulthood is an important clue with respect to pathophysiology because developmental changes may continue to occur in the brain during this period. The onset of the illness, with subsequent progression of symptoms during the first few years and later stabilization for the remaining years, makes schizophrenia very unusual among brain disorders. Given the complexity of this disorder, it is believed that progress may be facilitated by focusing on specific subgroups of patients with

This chapter was adapted from Nicolson R, Rapoport JL: Childhood-onset schizophrenia: what can it teach us?, in *Childhood Onset of "Adult" Psychopathology: Clinical and Research Advances.* Edited by Rapoport JL. Washington, DC, American Psychiatric Press, 2000, pp. 167–192 schizophrenia that seem to have an important unifying characteristic (Barondes et al. 1997).

Across medicine, the study of phenotypic extremes with an early onset has been an important approach to the understanding of disease (Tsuang et al. 2001). For example, unusually early onset of other multifactorial diseases, such as diabetes mellitus and rheumatoid arthritis, is associated with greater heritability and disease severity (Childs and Scriver 1986). Since 1990, a study of treatment-refractory childhood-onset schizophrenia (COS; onset of psychotic symptoms before age 12 years) has been ongoing at the National Institute of Mental Health (NIMH; Gordon et al. 1994b). The study of children with schizophrenia has been neglected because of the nosologic difficulties in defining the disorder in earlier DSM editions as well as its rarity. Although the treated prevalence has been reported to be 1/50 that of adult-onset schizophrenia (Beitchman 1985), this is almost certainly an overestimate given the high number of false-positive diagnoses inevitably included in such a survey (McKenna et al. 1994b).

Although rare, the study of early-onset schizophrenia may reveal important clues about the etiology of the disorder. The fact that this form of the disorder is often associated with severe illness has led to the speculation that early onset reflects a stronger biological predisposition, that it might represent a more genetically homogeneous form of the disorder, or both. Study of the factors that lead to the development of schizophrenia at an unusually early age may provide important clues about the timing and genetic basis of abnormal neural development leading to the emergence of schizophrenia. A better understanding of factors that trigger the onset of schizophrenia may lead to the development of novel therapeutic agents aimed at preventing schizophrenia's onset in vulnerable individuals.

This chapter reviews the evidence for continuity between COS and adult-onset schizophrenia. Preliminary data is presented that also suggest a similar pattern of associated risk factors between groups, along with evidence suggesting that COS may represent a more severe form of the disorder. Lastly, pharmacologic treatment studies using atypical neuroleptic agents in patients with neuroleptic-nonresponsive COS are also reviewed.

Is Childhood-Onset Schizophrenia Continuous With Adult-Onset Schizophrenia?

Studies at the NIMH and the University of California, Los Angeles (UCLA), have addressed the continuity question comprehensively (Asarnow et al.

1995; Gordon et al. 1994b; Jacobsen and Rapoport 1998; McKenna et al. 1994a). Examination of the phenomenology, neuropsychology, and biology of these patients has provided strong evidence that COS is clinically and biologically continuous with later-onset forms of the disorder.

Clinical Features

Several studies have demonstrated that schizophrenia can be reliably diagnosed in children using the same criteria as those applied to adults (Gordon et al. 1994b; Green et al. 1992; Kolvin 1971; Russell 1994; Spencer and Campbell 1994). Schizophrenia is rare in very young children, but its incidence rises sharply and steadily at about 12–14 years of age (Galdos et al. 1993; Hafner et al. 1993). The distinction between early-onset psychoses (before age 3) and later-onset psychoses (with onset at or after age 5) was one of the most important diagnostic advances in child psychiatry, separating autism from true childhood schizophrenia (Kolvin 1971). Later studies using populations defined by DSM-III (American Psychiatric Association 1980) and DSM-III-R (American Psychiatric Association 1987) have confirmed and extended these findings (Alaghband-Rad et al. 1995; Green et al. 1992; Russell 1994). COS is frequently insidious rather than acute in onset, and the most commonly reported psychotic features are auditory hallucinations and delusions (Green et al. 1992; Kolvin et al. 1971; Russell et al. 1994). The presence of formal thought disorder is more variable across studies and depends on the sample and the definition (Caplan 1994; Makowski et al. 1997).

Misdiagnosis of COS is common (McKenna et al. 1994) because of the overreliance on cross-sectional assessments or chart review (McClellan et al. 1993; Werry 1996), the variety of severe psychiatric disorders that overlap with COS (McKenna et al. 1994a, 1994b), and the limited experience of most clinicians in diagnosing the disorder. Cross-sectional diagnosis of children and adolescents with psychotic symptoms is problematic because there is considerable overlap in the presentation of first-episode bipolar disorder and schizophrenia (Werry 1996).

Multidimensionally Impaired Syndrome: Part of the Schizophrenia Spectrum?

The only way that the boundaries of the schizophrenia phenotype can be established with any certainty is through the use of some form of a diagnosis-specific biological marker. In the absence of good biological markers for schizophrenia, the exact boundaries of schizophrenia remain unclear. Although the categorical phenotype of schizophrenia using the

DSM classification system is important because these criteria demonstrate reliability, validity, and heritability, this may not be the nosology most relevant for identifying genetic loci given the problem of phenocopies, variable expressivity, and incomplete penetrance in complex inherited disorders (Gershon et al. 1998; Tsuang et al. 1998).

These difficulties in phenotypic definition have been highlighted in the study of autism. At first, it was considered unlikely that genetic factors played any major role in the etiology of the disorder because it was so uncommon to find more than one child in a family affected and because it was so exceedingly rare to find an autistic child with an autistic parent. However, when it was realized that the rate in siblings (2%) was much higher than the base rate in the general population (4 per 10,000), systematic twin studies were undertaken. Folstein and Rutter (1977a, 1977b) demonstrated that the concordance rate for certain cognitive and language disorders was 82% among monozygotic autistic twins and 10% among dizygotic autistic twins, suggesting that investigation of familial aggregation of a broader range of cognitive disorders was needed to define the phenotype in autism. Since then, observation of the relatives of autistic children has revealed that certain cognitive, social, language, and biochemical peculiarities may represent the variable expression of a gene or genes related to autism. A similar approach may aid in the clarification of the phenotypic boundaries of schizophrenia.

A sizable proportion of the children referred to the NIMH COS study who did not meet criteria for schizophrenia were those with histories of transient psychotic symptoms in addition to disruptive behaviors and learning deficits. These children have been described by our group as multidimensionally impaired (MDI; Kumra et al. 1998a); however, children with a similar constellation of perceptual disturbances, cognitive deficits, and behavior problems have been described as having multiplex developmental disorder (Towbin et al. 1993) or being borderline (Kernberg 1990). Self-reported psychotic symptoms in prepubertal children appear to be a strong childhood risk factor for the development of adult schizophreniform disorder (Poulton et al. 2000). These data suggest that it might be possible to screen for children at risk for psychosis, which would allow for a better description of the neural substrate of schizophrenia prior to illness onset and of the impact of environmental adversity for subsequent psychosis. Furthermore, clarifying the connections between children with narrowly defined schizophrenia and children with a more broadly defined phenotype (i.e., MDI) has implications for understanding the pathophysiology of schizophrenia.

Both the MDI and COS patients shared a similar pattern of premorbid developmental difficulties, cognitive deficits, a diminution in cognitive ability from a higher premorbid level, magnetic resonance imaging (MRI) abnormalities, cytogenetic abnormalities, and increased rates of schizophrenia spectrum disorders in first-degree relatives (Kumra et al. 1998a, 1998c, 2000a).

In contrast to patients with COS, the MDI cohort had an overrepresentation of male subjects, earlier cognitive and behavior difficulties, earlier age of onset of psychotic symptoms, a more striking depression in the freedom from distractability factor on the Wechsler Intelligence Scale for Children–Revised (WISC-R), and a less deviant pattern of autonomic activity. These distinguishing features support our initial phenomenologic distinction of these cases from COS.

Although these data distinguished MDI children from children with other psychiatric disorders, it remains unclear whether MDI should be conceptualized as an alternate expression of COS or a variant of some other disorder. Some of the children with MDI appear to be at risk for developing more severe chronic psychotic disorders because preliminary 2- to 4-year follow-up data have shown that 4 (21%) of 19 patients have gone on to develop schizoaffective disorder, bipolar type.

Children and adolescents with MDI have a similar pattern of premorbid developmental disturbances as children with schizophrenia and resemble them in a number of biological parameters (Kumra et al. 1998c). Assuming that schizophrenia is caused by several allelic variations of normal genes that function by increasing or decreasing susceptibility to environmental stressors, then the phenomenologic similarities between multidimensional impairment and COS could reflect overlapping or shared etiologic factors between the two disorders that result in a disruption of brain development. The MDI group may allow more ambitious genetic studies, as it is larger than the narrow band of patients with COS.

Neurobiological Studies

Neurobiological studies of patients with COS have supported a hypothesis that COS is continuous with the later-onset disorder. These include neuropsychological impairments, structural brain MRI abnormalities, proton MRI abnormalities, and eye tracking dysfunction (Table 7–1).

Neuropsychology

Numerous studies have shown that whereas cognitive deficits, particularly in the areas of attention, verbal learning, and executive functions, are

Table 7–1. Childhood-onset schizophrenia: continuity with adult-onset schizophrenia

Measure	Continuity	Resemblance to adults with poor outcome	Reference
Clinical presentation	+ (by definition)	+	Gordon et al. 1994b McKenna et al. 1994b
Premorbid function	+	+	Alaghband-Rad et al. 1995 Hollis 1995
Neuropsychology	+	+	R. F. Asarnow et al. 1994 Kumra et al. 2000b
Autonomic functioning	+	+	Zahn et al. 1997
SPEM abnormalites	+	+	Jacobsen et al. 1996a Kumra et al. in press
Anatomic brain MRI	+	+	Frazier et al. 1996 Jacobsen et al. 1996a, 1997b, 1997c, 1997d
PET	+	–	Jacobsen et al. 1997a
MRS	+	?	Bertolino et al. 1998

Note. MRI=magnetic resonance imaging; MRS=magnetic resonance spectroscopy; PET=positron emission tomography; SPEM=smooth pursuit eye movement.

present in most patients with schizophrenia (COS and later-onset schizophrenia), single-word oral reading ability is relatively preserved (Asarnow et al. 1995; Frith 1996; Paulsen et al. 1995). The neuropsychological test results for the NIMH COS group were 1–2 standard deviations below normative data across a broad array of cognitive functions, perhaps reflecting limited information-processing capacity (Kumra et al. 2000b). Neuroleptic-nonresponsive COS subjects showed a similar pattern of generalized cognitive deficits on the same type of tasks (e.g., Wisconsin Card Sorting Test [WCST]; Rey-Osterreith Complex Figure direct copy; Trail Making A and B; Digit, Digit Symbol, Verbal Learning subtests of the Wide Range Assessment of Memory and Learning [WRAML]) that detect impairments in patients with later-onset schizophrenia (Bilder et al. 2000; Braff 1991; Kenny et al. 1997; Saykin et al. 1994) and other patients with

COS (R.F. Asarnow et al. 1994). A pattern of cognitive deficits in verbal and visual memory and auditory attention similar to that observed in our COS cohort has also been reported in the relatives and offspring of patients with schizophrenia (Asarnow et. al. 1977; Kremen et al. 1998) and in first-episode, neuroleptic-naïve patients (Nopoulos et al. 1998; Saykin et al. 1994). Thus, the observed findings are not likely to be the result of psychotic process or even secondary effects of psychosis on cognitive development. Knowing a child's neuropsychological impairments and assets can be helpful for treatment planning. Certain forms of memory or vigilance deficits may hinder a child's psychosocial adjustment and academic success; for this reason, these deficits should be considered targets for intervention and remediation. Longtudinal studies of both childhood (Bedwell et al. 1999) and adult-onset schizophrenic patients (Heaton et al. 2001) support the view that neuropsychological deficits in schizophrenia are stable, trait-like dimensions of the disorder and provide no evidence of a deteriorating neuropsychological course.

Magnetic Resonance Imaging

It has been assumed that the structural brain abnormalities seen in patients with schizophrenia reflect the influence of factors contributing to disease susceptibility. However, no structural MRI abnormality has been consistently found in all affected individuals diagnosed with COS, and for each measure considerable overlap exists between patients and healthy control subjects (Frazier et al. 1996; Table 7–2).

In addition, earlier age at onset of psychotic symptoms does not appear to be related to the degree of brain dysmorphology (e.g., deficit in cortical gray matter volume and enlargement of cortical sulcal and ventricular cerebrospinal fluid volumes compared with age-matched normal control subjects) in adults with schizophrenia (Lim et al. 1996).

MRI abnormalities of brain morphology have been repeatedly observed in adults with schizophrenia (Shenton et al. 1997), and those with COS have been found to have similar abnormalities (Frazier er al.1996; Jacobsen et al. 1997b, 1997c). Analyses of the scans of 35 COS patients and 57 matched control subjects (see Table 7–2) show the expected increase in lateral ventricular volume with decreased cerebellar volume and midsagittal thalamic area. It is of interest, however, that reductions in the volumes of the anterior frontal lobes and medial temporal lobes (Frazier et al. 1996; Jacobsen et al. 1996b, 1997d) were not found in the patients with COS. Using a different methodology, these results recently have been replicated in a separate group of children and adolescents with

Table 7–2. Magnetic resonance imaging brain anatomy in childhood-onset schizophrenia

Measure	ANOVA		ANCOVA*		Comment
	F	**P**	**F**	**P**	
Total cerebral volume	1.53	0.13			
White matter	0.00	0.98	29.00	0.0001	COS>NC
Gray matter	9.98	0.002	45.00	0.0001	COS<NC
Prefrontal	4.42	0.04	2.65	0.11	
Corpus callosum	1.36	0.25	5.02	0.30	COS>NC
Lateral ventricles	8.47	0.004	9.33	0.003	COS>NC
Ventricle-to-brain ratio	3.23	0.002			COS>NC
Temporal lobe	0.19	0.66	0.20	0.66	Subdivisions also not significantly different Planum temporale asymmetry not different between COS and NC
Hippocampus	3.74	0.565	2.10	0.15	NC: R>L COS: R=L
Amygdala	2.86	0.09	0.77	0.38	NC: R>L COS: R>L
Cerebellum	9.71	0.003	7.56	0.008	COS<NC COS had decreased midsagittal vermal area and inferior posterior lobe (VIII-X)
Thalamus (area)	4.81	<0.0001	16.50	0.0001	COS<NC

Note. *ANCOVA covaried for total brain volume; all *P* values two-tailed.
ANOVA=analysis of variance; ANCOVA=analysis of covariance; COS=childhood-onset schizophrenia (*n*=35); NC=normal control subjects (*n*=57); L=left; R=right.

early-onset schizophrenia; however, in that study, localization of enlarged ventricles was specific to the posterior region (Sowell et al. 2000).

A recent meta-analysis found a significant association between schizophrenia and bilateral volumetric reduction of the hippocampus (Nelson et al. 1998). Although we did not find volume reductions in medial temporal lobe structures in patients with COS, similar negative findings have been reported for other early-onset patients with schizophrenia (Matsumodo et al. 2001) and adults with early-onset schizophrenia (Marsh et al. 1997). Of interest, pilot data suggest that structural brain abnormalities of the medial temporal lobe may be a late-developing phenomenon (Jacobsen et al. 1998).

Studies have suggested that the maldeveloped neural circuitry producing schizophrenic symptoms may include the cerebellum. Subnormal activation of prefrontal–thalamic–cerebellar circuitry has been demonstrated in unmedicated adults with schizophrenia performing practiced and novel memory tasks, suggesting that cognitive dysmetria or poor cordination of retrieval, processing, and expression of information may be fundamental deficits in patients with schizophrenia (Andreasen et al. 1998). To test this hypothesis, anatomic brain scans were acquired with a 1.5-T MRI scanner for 24 patients (mean age, 14.1 years; SD=2.2) with onset of schizophrenia by age 12 (mean age at onset, 10.0 years; SD=1.9) and 52 healthy children. After adjustment for total cerebral volume, the volumes of the vermis, midsagittal area, and inferior posterior lobe of the cerebellum remained significantly smaller in the patients with schizophrenia (Jacobsen et al. 1997c). These findings are consistent with observations of small vermal size in adult schizophrenia and provide further support for abnormal cerebellar function in COS and adult-onset schizophrenia (Jacobsen et al. 1997c).

The planum temporale has been linked to language processing and schizophrenic pathology. The planum temporale shows a prominent leftward (left greater than right) asymmetry in 70% of healthy individuals. In a study of 16 adolescent patients with COS, no differences between healthy adolescents and those with schizophrenia in the planum temporale area or asymmetry were observed. However, post-hoc analyses revealed that within the group of patients with schizophrenia, a history of prepsychotic language disorder was associated with abnormal asymmetry (rightwardly asymmetric or symmetric). These findings do not support a hypothesis for anomalous planum temporale asymmetry as a basis for psychopathology in patients with COS (Jacobsen et al. 1997d).

Patients with COS were found to have increased rates of a developmental brain anomaly—enlarged cavum septi pellucidi (CSP)—compared with healthy subjects: 3 (12.5%) of 24 patients had the anomaly versus 1 (1.1%) of 95 healthy subjects. Although the rate of CSP enlargement is very similar to what has been reported in studies of adult patients, two patients were found to have a combined cavum septi pellucidi and cavum vergum, which represents a more severe lack of fusion of the septal leaflets (Noupolos et al. 1998). CSP can be considered a midline neurodevelopmental anomaly involving a limbic structure. The presence of CSP is most likely indirectly related to the underlying pathology of schizophrenia.

A magnetic resonance spectroscopy study of patients with COS revealed decreases in the N-acetylaspartate (NAA)-to-creatine ratio, a putative marker of neuronal integrity, exclusively in the prefrontal cortex and hippocampus (Bertolino et al. 1998). No correlation was found between NAA measures in the hippocampal area and dorsolateral prefrontal cortex and the volume of these structures as measured by MRI, suggesting that they are not related to volumetric losses. These results are consistent both in extent and location of the damage with earlier findings from patients with adult-onset schizophrenia that showed low NAA values in the mesial temporal-limbic and prefrontal cortices (Bertolino et al. 1998); however, interpretation of the NAA finding is controversial, because other investigators have failed to find lower NAA levels in patients with schizophrenia (Bartha et al. 1997). Patients with COS did not have more severe hippocampal abnormalities compared with adult patients.

Neurophysiological Studies

Abnormalities in peripheral indicators of autonomic activity (e.g., skin conductance and heart rate) have been noted in those with adult-onset schizophrenia. In patients with COS, a striking hyporesponsivity in skin conductance responses to both novel and significant stimuli has been observed; this appears to be related to the severity of both positive and negative symptoms of schizophrenia. A study of autonomic functioning in patients with COS (Zahn et al. 1997) found them comparable on this measure to adults with chronic, poor-outcome schizophrenia.

Smooth Pursuit Eye Movements

From 40% to 80% of patients with adult-onset schizophrenia have abnormalities in smooth pursuit eye movements (SPEMs; Levy et al. 1993). The finding of similar abnormalities in 30%–50% of the biological first-degree relatives of probands with schizophrenia and in the offspring of schizophrenic parents suggests that this may be a genetic marker of vulnerability to the illness (Levy et al. 1993). The higher rate of eye tracking dysfunction as compared with disease phenotype of schizophrenia in the first-degree relatives of patients with schizophrenia suggests that this may be a useful trait to increase the power of genetic studies. Patients with COS have abnormalities similar to those reported in adult patients: poorer global qualitative ratings, decreased gain (ratio of eye speed to target speed), increased root mean square error (global indicator of aberrant tracking), and increased anticipatory saccades compared with healthy subjects (Jacobsen et al. 1996a; Kumra et al. in press). Genetic high risk studies will be instructive to understand the normal developmental course of SPEM in childhood and the relationship between SPEM and behavioral abnormalities.

In summary, the NIMH study supports clinical and biological continuity between COS and adult-onset schizophrenia. It is theoretically possible, however, that COS and later-onset schizophrenia may have a different pathogenesis, with similar biological markers reflecting a final common pathway. Ongoing studies are relating these neurobiological abnormalities in COS to various familial risk factors. A second issue is to establish the nature of the underlying pathology. It should be stressed that the observed MRI abnormalities do not indicate a site of the pathogenic process involved in COS; experimental approaches are needed to test hypotheses on the links between structure and function. The next level of structural MRI studies will require integration with other in vivo modalities such as diffusion tensor imaging and functional MRI to provide greater insight into the core pathophysiology of early-onset schizophrenia (Giedd 2001).

Is Childhood-Onset Schizophrenia A More Severe Form of the Disorder?

The notable differences between COS and later-onset schizophrenia are in the areas of genetic loading, frequency of cytogenetic abnormalities, premorbid development, clinical outcome, and longitudinal brain imaging studies.

Genetic Factors

Genetic factors are thought to play a major role in the pathogenesis of schizophrenia (Karayiorgou and Gogos 1997), and the possibility of a single locus with a very large effect (a Mendelian-type gene) operating in COS led to two classic studies (Kallmann and Roth 1956; Kolvin 1971).

Age at onset in schizophrenia has a lower correlation between affected siblings (approximately 0.26) and concordant dizygotic twins (approximately 0.30) than between concordant monozygotic twins (mean, 0.68; Kendler et al. 1987), suggesting genetic influences on age at onset. However, the lack of relationship between pedigree density and age at onset in most studies (Kendler et al. 1987, 1996) suggests that age at onset is influenced by genetic factors that are unrelated to the disease liability. Additionally, the correlation of less than 1.0 in monozygotic twins suggests a role for nongenetic factors in determining age at onset. As with most studies, those reviewed by Kendler did not include COS populations. Thus, there remains the possibility that very-early-onset cases may reveal more unique or potent genetic factors.

Schizophrenia and spectrum disorders (i.e., schizoaffective disorder and schizotypal and paranoid personality disorders) are increased in the relatives of patients with schizophrenia (Kendler et al. 1993a, 1993b, 1993c). Adoption studies (Kendler et al. 1994) document the genetic basis for these spectrum disorders. Previous studies of COS (Kallman and Roth 1956; Kolvin 1971) found a twofold increase in the aggregation of schizophrenic disorders among the first-degree relatives of patients of COS compared with adult-onset cases. However, these studies did not include unblinded assessments, control groups, structured diagnostic instruments, or operationalized diagnostic criteria, all of which may have biased the results.

First-degree relatives in the NIMH cohort were administered either the Diagnostic Interview for Children and Adolescents (in relatives younger than age 18 years) or the children's version of the Schedule for Affective Disorders and Schizophrenia (SADS; Orvaschel et al. 1980). Relatives older than age 17 years were administered the SADS and the Structured Interview for DSM-III-R or DSM-IV Personality Disorders (SID-P). Three (3.3%) of 92 first-degree relatives were determined to have schizophrenia, and 23 (25%) of 92 available first-degree relatives were found to have either paranoid or schizotypal personality disorder (M. Lenane, unpublished data, 1999). Similar elevated rates of schizophrenic spectrum disorders in the first-degree relatives of COS probands have also been reported in a less severely ill cohort in a recent, methodologically rigorous family study of COS probands (Asarnow et al. 2001). In relatives of individuals with adult-onset schizophrenia, the rate of schizotypal personality disorder was found to be 6.9% and the rate of paranoid personality disorder was found to be 1.4% (Kendler et al. 1993a, 1993b, 1993c; Table 7–3).

Although the rates of schizophrenia and schizoaffective disorder in relatives of COS patients are similar to those seen in relatives of adult-

Table 7–3. Rates of schizophrenia spectrum disorders in first-degree relatives of patients with childhood-onset schizophrenia (NIMH sample), relatives of adult patients with adult-onset schizophrenia (published family data), and relatives of nonschizophrenic adult control subjects (family data)

Diagnosis	Relatives of patients with childhood-onset schizophrenia	Relatives of patients with adult-onset schizophrenia,* %	Relatives of nonschizophrenic control subjects,* %
Schizophrenia	3/92 (3.3%)	6.5	0.5
Schizoaffective disorder	1/89 (1.1%)	2.3	0.7
Schizotypal personality disorder	10/90 (11.1%)	6.9	1.4
Paranoid personality disorder	9/80 (11.3%)	1.4	0.4
Relatives with schizophrenia spectrum disorder	23/92 (25.0%)		
Patients with a relative with schizophrenia or a spectrum disorder	18/40 (45.0%)		

Note. Rates determined using hierarchical method (Kendler 1988).
*Kendler et al. 1993a, 1993b, 1993c

onset patients, there appears to be an excess of schizotypal and paranoid personality disorders in those with COS. However, these results must be interpreted with great caution because direct comparison of rates of disorder in relatives of childhood-onset and adult-onset schizophrenia probands diagnosed by identical methods is required before firm conclusions about differential aggregation can be reached (Asarnow et al. 2001). These preliminary data nonetheless suggest a more salient role for genetic factors in these very-early-onset patients.

Spectrum disorders in first-degree relatives were powerfully related to premorbid abnormalities in our patients with COS. Thirteen (72%) of the patients with relatives with schizophrenia or spectrum disorders had premorbid language abnormalities, but only seven (32%) without a similar family history had early language difficulties ($P=0.006$).

Another indirect measure of genetic risk for schizophrenia is SPEMs, which have been proposed as a marker of liability to schizophrenia in unaffected relatives of probands (Levy et al. 1993). To date, 52 relatives of our probands have been examined and, using the root mean square error, 13 were determined to have abnormal eye tracking. These abnormalities appear to be similar in frequency to those seen in the relatives of adult-onset patients (Rapoport and Inoff-Germain 2000).

Chromosomal Abnormalities

Historically, chromosomal abnormalities have sometimes provided information helpful in the localization of disease-susceptibility loci. In adults with schizophrenia, an increased rate of sex chromosome abnormalities has been reported (DeLisi et al. 1994), and other chromosomal abnormalities have been observed less consistently (Bassett 1992; Karayiorgou and Gogos 1997). To date, 3 (6.4%) of 47 COS patients were found to have a 22q11 deletion. All 3 had premorbid impairments of language, motor, and social development, although their physical characteristics varied (Usiskin et al. 1999). Of the genes mapped to 22q11, a common functional polymorphism of catecho-O-methyltransferase may be a candidate gene for schizophrenia (Egan et al. 2001). This functional variant increases prefrontal catabolism, which results in impaired prefrontal cognition and physiology (Egan et al. 2001). Two additional COS patients in this series were also noted to have cytogenic abnormalities that include a Turner's mosaic; mos46, X, del[X][q24][47]/45,X[3]; female; and a boy with translocation of chromosomes 1 and 7. An additional three sex chromosome abnormalities (two Klinefelter's [XXY] and one XYY) occurred in 28 MDI patients (Kumra et al. 1998a). The process by which either sex chromosome abnormalities or deletions of chromosome 22q11 lead to the development of psychotic disorders is unknown. The question of whether patients with sex chromosome aneuploidies have an increased frequency of schizophrenia or schizophrenia-like symptoms is now being studied in unselected populations (i.e., a birth cohort in which all infants identified with these genetic abnormalities at birth will be followed prospectively). Preliminary findings from one such study do not support a relationship between sex chromosome aneuploidies and schizophrenia (Mors et al. 2001).

Premorbid Features

Follow-back studies suggest that prodromal symptoms of COS may include developmental delays, disruptive behavior disorders, expressive and receptive language deficits, impaired gross motor functioning, learning and academic problems, full-scale IQ in the borderline to low average range, and transient symptoms of pervasive developmental disorder (Alaghband-Rad et al. 1995; Russell et al. 1994; Watkins et al. 1988; Werry et al. 1991). Although similar premorbid abnormalities have been observed in patients with adult-onset schizophrenia (Parnas et al. 1982; Walker et al. 1990), the rate of language impairments and transient autistic-like and nonspecific symptoms appears higher in those with COS (Hafner and Nowonty 1995; Hollis 1995).

Although these data are supportive of a hypothesis that a more severe early disruption of brain development is associated with COS, these prodromal symptoms may not be direct manifestations of the schizophrenic diathesis; rather, they may be nonspecific signs of a vulnerability associated with increased risk for a variety of disorders.

An updated analysis of the prepsychotic developmental data (i.e., school and medical reports, previous psychological and language testing) of 41 patients with COS studied at the NIMH confirms the findings of previous studies. To date, 44% of the patients had social abnormalities, 49% had language abnormalities, and 32% had motor abnormalities years before the onset of psychotic symptoms. About 50% had transient premorbid behavioral and language symptoms resembling those seen in autistic disorder (Alaghband-Rad et al. 1995). Because the patients in the NIMH study were selected for poor treatment response, a comparison with unselected adult-onset schizophrenic patients may not be entirely appropriate, and ongoing studies are addressing this. Similarly, retrospective adult data cannot be strictly compared with these data because of a lack of blinding and different age of the historical material.

The most common communication difficulties in patients with COS have been reported in the area of pragmatics (i.e., referencing the listener, establishing topics of discourse, sequencing events, taking turns), prosody, auditory processing, and expressive and receptive language (Baltaxe and Simmons 1995). Of note, the recent localization of a gene implicated in severe speech and language disorders to chromosome 7q31 may be a potential candidate gene for the linguistic abnormalities observed in patients with COS (Lai et al. 2000). It is unknown whether any of the linguistic abnormalities reported in COS probands are exhibited in their first-degree relatives (Baltaxe and Simmons 1995).

Clinical Outcome

The outcome of patients with COS is generally thought to be poor and possibly worse than that of the adult-onset cases (Hollis 2000). Three studies that examined outcome after an average interval of about 5 years have reported rates of remission ranging from 3% (Werry et al. 1991) to 30% (J.R. Asarnow et al. 1994; Russell 1994). Schmidt et al. (1995) examined the clinical and social outcome of COS patients (defined as age of onset younger than 18 years) compared with that of adult-onset patients after a mean follow-up period of 7.4 years. They found that more than two-thirds of the 118 patients in their sample had had at least one further schizophrenic episode and were in need of continuing psychiatric treatment. Social impairment was greater for the COS patients, particularly in the areas of self-care and social contacts. In two studies (Maziade et al 1996) with longer follow-up periods (average, 15–16 years), the reported rates of full remission were 5% and 20%, respectively, with most patients experiencing continuing symptoms.

Eggers and Bunk (1997) have reported the longest follow-up data (i.e., 42 years) on a small sample ($n = 44$) of early-onset cases. They found that 50% of the patients had continuous symptoms and 25% were in partial remission. Abnormal premorbid adjustment, insidious mode of onset of psychotic symptoms, and onset of psychotic symptoms before age 12 appear to be the best predictors of poor clinical outcome (Amminger et al. 1997; Eggers and Bunk 1997; Werry and McClellan 1992). Together, these studies suggest that the care of patients with COS requires significant resource utilization and that conventional neuroleptic agents have limited effects with regard to the long-term morbidity associated with COS.

Longitudinal Magnetic Resonance Imaging Studies

It is known that the human brain undergoes significant anatomic and metabolic changes during adolescence (Chugani et al. 1996; Huttenlocher 1979), and these changes have been suggested as fundamental to the development of schizophrenia (Feinberg 1982–1983). A prospective longitudinal study of anatomic brain changes as measured by MRI scans has been an integral component of the NIMH study of COS patients.

Although progressive changes in the brains of adult patients with schizophrenia have been reported (DeLisi et al. 1995; Gur et al. 1998; Lieberman et al. 1996), patients with COS appear to have a differential enlargement of the lateral ventricles and cortical gray matter that is more marked and consistent compared with what has been reported previously for adult-onset patients (Rapoport et al. 1997, 1999). Although brain changes have been noted after treatment with antipsychotic agents (Chakos et al. 1995; Frazier et al. 1996), the differential progression observed in these patients is not consistent with the reported effects of antipsychotic medications on brain structure. Despite the progressive ventricular enlargement in the COS patients, there is no evidence of true cognitive deterioration. Temporal lobe developmental progression may have a similar late component. Pilot data indicate a differential progression with greater hippocampal decrease in patients with very-early-onset schizophrenia (Jacobsen et al. 1998).

In contrast, MRI studies of brain development in healthy children demonstrate very subtle linear progressive changes in lateral ventricular volume starting in the first decade of life (Giedd et al. 1999). This slight ventricular volume increase is not tightly linked to puberty and thus does not typically change during the years before the usual onset of schizophrenia.

Atypical Neuroleptic Agents in the Treatment of Neuroleptic-Nonresponsive Childhood-Onset Schizophrenia

Although there are compelling controlled trial data to support the use of antipsychotic agents in patients with psychotic disorders, there have been few studies in patients younger than age 18 years. Nonetheless, existing data suggest that apart from differences in titration schedule, dosing, and side effects, treatment response would appear to be similar in both adult-onset and childhood-onset patients (Campbell and Cueva 1995a, 1995b). Short-term efficacy has been generally measured by reductions in positive or negative symptoms among treated patients during 4–8-week medication trials. An advantage of these studies is that they clearly demonstrate how well a medication can reduce target symptoms, but what is less clear is whether symptomatic improvement will lead to substantial improvements in long-term outcome.

Approximately 70% of patients with schizophrenia receive some benefit from typical neuroleptic agents (i.e., reduction in the severity of hallucinations and delusions); however, it is estimated that only 40% of patients experience good recovery in social functioning (Conley and Buchanan 1997; Marder 1999; Maziade et al. 1996). Although it is uncertain whether children and adolescents with schizophrenia are actually less responsive to neuroleptic agents (Pool et al. 1976; Spencer et al. 1992), earlier age of onset in adult patients is reported to be a predictor of poor therapeutic response (Lieberman et al. 1996; Pickar et al. 1993).

In the United States, 30 children and adolescents with schizophrenia who have shown poor responses to treatment have been studied at the NIMH in either open or double-blind protocols. The NIMH cohort of neuroleptic-nonresponsive schizophrenic patients is characterized by an equal distribution of males and females, with approximately two-thirds of the patients having an insidious onset of their disorder. At the time of referral, many of the patients had already had periods of hospitalization as well as considerable exposure to antipsychotic medications (Kumra et al. 1996).

A double-blind parallel comparison of haloperidol and clozapine in 21 treatment-refractory COS patients (all with onset of psychotic symptoms before age 12; mean age, 14.0 years) found clozapine superior to haloperidol for both positive and negative symptoms and for measures of overall improvement (Kumra et al. 1996). Clozapine dosages began at 6.25–25 mg/day, depending on the patient's weight, and could be increased every 3–4 days by one to two times the starting dosage on an individual basis. The mean dosage of clozapine at week 6 of treatment was 149 mg/day (range, 25–525 mg/day). Medical monitoring included weekly complete blood cell counts with differential, liver function tests, an encephalogram, and an electrocardiogram before drug initiation and at week 6 of treatment. Patients who were initially randomized to the haloperidol treatment arm of the study received a 6-week open-label trial of clozapine.

At the completion of this 6-week clozapine trial, many COS patients were able to return to a less restrictive setting because of the dramatic improvement in clinical symptoms and reduction of aggressive outbursts associated with clozapine treatment. Thirteen of 21 patients who participated in the double-blind trial continued taking clozapine for an additional 30–45 months after completion of the study, and continued benefits in overall functioning have been seen at the 2-year follow-up examination (Kumra S., Jacobsen L.K., unpublished data, 1998).

Unfortunately, as seen in adults, the use of clozapine may be associated with serious adverse events such as blood dyscrasias and seizures. In the NIMH sample, 7 of 27 patients had to stop otherwise effective clozapine therapy because of serious adverse events: two of these patients developed neutropenias (absolute neutrophil count less than 1,500), which recurred with drug rechallenge; three patients developed persistent seizure activity despite anticonvulsant treatment; one patient developed excessive weight gain; and one patient developed a threefold elevation in liver enzymes. In each of these cases, there were no permanent or long-lasting negative consequences after drug withdrawal.

Similar findings were reported by Turetz et al. (1997) in 11 children with treatment-resistant schizophrenia who were treated with clozapine in an open-label study. Treatment response was monitored using the Brief Psychiatric Rating Scale (BPRS), Positive and Negative Syndrome Scale (PANSS), and Clinical Global Impressions (CGI) scale over a 16-week period. The patients' clinical conditions showed an overall improvement, mostly within the first 6–8 weeks, that was greater for positive symptoms. Somnolence and hypersalivation were the most serious side effects, and there were no incidents of agranulocytosis.

Ten children with treatment-refractory schizophrenia from the NIMH cohort were also treated with olanzapine in either open or double-blind trials (Kumra et al. 1998b). Some of the patients included in this trial were intolerant of clozapine but had been good responders to the drug. Compared with the side effect data collected from patients treated with clozapine at our center, olanzapine has been well tolerated in this group using dosages up to 20 mg/day. For this protocol, olanzapine dosages were initiated at 2.5 mg every other day (weight less than 40 kg) or 2.5 mg/day (weight above 40 kg), depending on the child's weight. Dosages could be increased to 2.5 mg/day (weight less than 40 kg) or 5 mg/day (weight above 40 kg) on day 3. Thereafter, the dosage was adjusted upward to a maximum of 20 mg/day (using day 1 of treatment as the start date) by 2.5–5 mg every 5–9 days as determined by the treating physician. The CGI scale was used to assess improvement after 8 weeks on olanzapine compared with the clinical condition on entry into the study. To date, of the 10 patients who participated in this trial, three were rated "much improved," four were "minimally improved," one had "no change," one was "minimally worse," and one was "much worse" (Kumra et al. 1998b). The mean dosage of medication at week 6 of treatment with olanzapine was 17.5 ± 2.3 mg/day (range, 12.5–20 mg). The most frequent side effects included increased appetite, constipation, nausea or vomiting, headache, somnolence, insomnia, difficulty concentrating, sustained tachycardia, increased nervousness, and transient elevation of liver transaminases. The incidence of these minor side effects is comparable with the side effect profile of patients who have participated in open or double-blind trials of clozapine. No cases of neutropenia or seizures have occurred with olanzapine.

Although olanzapine has a more benign side effect profile than clozapine, preliminary data based on a comparison of 23 patients who received 6-week open trials of clozapine, olanzapine, or both at the NIMH show that clozapine has superior efficacy for both positive and negative symptoms for this group of severely ill children (Kumra et al. 1998b). In addition, four patients who were responsive to clozapine but who could not continue on the drug because of serious adverse events received an open trial of olanzapine after having received a double-blind trial of clozapine. For this group, each patient was less symptomatic (as measured by the BPRS total score) at week 6 of clozapine treatment compared with olanzapine ($P = 0.03$; Kumra et al. 1998b).

The results of this comparison should be considered preliminary because of the small number of patients studied, lack of randomization, open-label design, fixed order of drug trials (most patients received a trial of clozapine first), and limitations of comparing open-label with double-blind data. However, based on these preliminary data, we have initiated an 8-week double-blind comparison trial of clozapine and olanzapine to directly evaluate the relative safety and efficacy of these treatments. The examination of the factors related to positive drug response in patients should be examined in the future.

Conclusions

Morphometric analyses of the brains of adult patients with schizophrenia have revealed a profile of increased neuronal density in the prefrontal and occipital cortices of patients relative to healthy comparison subjects (Selemon and Goldman-Rakic 1999). It has been hypothesized that the increased neuronal density in the prefrontal cortex of schizophrenic brains (which suggests a deficit in neuronal connections) may underlie the cognitive dysfunction seen in schizophrenic patients (Selemon and Goldman-Rakic 1999). Given the growing evidence for the plasticity of neurons in adult mammalian brains, there is a possibility that treatments may be developed in the future for remodeling neuronal processes, assuming that cortical neurons are preserved in those with schizophrenia. Based on this hypothesis, there has been a push to identify individuals who are at an early stage of transition to frank psychosis or to identify genetic markers with high predictive validity for the development of schizophrenia. It has been proposed that early treatment with either psychosocial interventions or antipsychotic medication could prevent the onset of psychosis or minimize the morbidity associated with a first episode of a psychotic disorder. However, other psychotropic medications with putative neuroprotective properties (Anand et al. 2000; Moore et al. 2000) may be effective, and phase-specific pharmacological interventions also may be required (Cornblatt et al. 1998).

The initial phase of the NIMH study has demonstrated convincing evidence for clinical and biological continuity between the very-early-onset and adult-onset forms of the disorder. Data from the NIMH COS study will be informative to researchers studying adolescents who are at genetic or clinical high risk for developing schizophrenia. Findings from the project have provided insight into a variety of risk factors and biological markers associated with the disorder that can be detected during adolescence as well as aberrant neurodevelopmental processes that may only be seen during adolescence in patients with schizophrenia. In addition, important treatment data supporting the utility of the atypical neuroleptic agents for children and adolescents with schizophrenia have emerged from the project.

The focus of the NIMH COS study has now turned to the potentially more important question of why these children have an earlier age of onset. In investigating potential causes, it appears that patients with COS have more severe premorbid abnormalities, more cytogenetic abnormalities, and potentially greater family histories. Although these data have several limitations, including probable selection bias for more severe cases from more research-compliant families, the pattern of our findings is suggestive of a greater genetic vulnerability in COS that may result in the earlier development of symptoms. Studies aimed at identifying potential susceptibility genes for schizophrenia in this group, integrating both clinical and neurobiological data, are currently in progress. The inclusion of the MDI patients, who share some phenomenological similarities with the COS patients, may allow for more ambitious genetic studies.

The association between spectrum disorders in the relatives of probands and speech and language abnormalities in our patients is of interest. The British birth cohort studies (Jones and Done 1997) both found speech and motor development in infancy and speech difficulties and word pronunciation at ages 7 and 11 years to be predictive of a later onset of schizophrenia. Additional studies examining the frequency and nature of speech and language difficulties in relatives of COS patients are warranted and may reveal that these traits have a higher genetic signal than the categorical phenotype of schizophrenia.

The cytogenetic and clinical findings suggest that even more intense screening of the X chromosome (DeLisi et al. 2000; Paterson 1999; Toniolo and D'Adamo 2000) and chromosome 7 (Barrett et al. 1999; Folstein and Mankoski 2000; Warburton et al. 2000) would be relevant given the relatively low IQ, premorbid linguistic abnormalities, and autistic-like features in a significant proportion of our cohort. Such studies are ongoing.

References

Alaghband-Rad J, McKenna K, Gordon CT, et al: Childhood-onset schizophrenia: the severity of premorbid course. J Am Acad Child Adolesc Psychiatry 34:1273–1283, 1995

American Psychiatric Association: Diagnostic and Statistical Manual of Mental Disorders, 3rd Edition. Washington, DC, American Psychiatric Association, 1980

American Psychiatric Association: Diagnostic and Statistical Manual of Mental Disorders, 3rd Edition Revised. Washington, DC, American Psychiatric Association, 1987

Amminger GP, Resch F, Mutschlechner R, et al: Premorbid adjustment and remission of positive symptoms in first-episode psychosis. Eur Child Adolesc Psychiatry 6:212–218, 1997

Anand A, Charney DS, Oren DA, et al: Attenuation of the neuropsychiatric effects of ketamine with lamotrigine: support for hyperglutamatergic effects of N-methyl-D-aspartate receptor antagonists. Arch Gen Psychiatry 57:270–276, 2000

Andreasen NC, Paradiso S, O'Leary DS: "Cognitive dysmetria" as an integrative theory of schizophrenia: a dysfunction in cortical-subcortical-cerebellar circuitry? Schizophr Bull 24:203–218, 1998

Asarnow JR, Tompson MC, Goldstein MJ: Childhood-onset schizophrenia: a follow-up study. Schizophr Bull 20:599–617, 1994

Asarnow RF, Steffy RA, MacCrimmon DJ, et al: An attentional assessment of foster children at risk for schizophrenia. J Abnorm Psychol 86:267–275, 1977

Asarnow RF, Asamen J, Granholm E, et al: Cognitive/neuropsychological studies of children with a schizophrenic disorder. Schizophr Bull 20:647–669, 1994

Asarnow RF, Brown W, Strandburg R: Children with a schizophrenic disorder: neurobehavioral studies. Eur Arch Psychiatry Clin Neurosci 245:70–79, 1995

Baltaxe AM, Simmons III JQ: Speech and language disorders in children and adolescents with schizophrenia. Schizophr Bull 21:677–692, 1995

Barondes SH, Alberts BM, Andreasen NC, et al: Workshop on schizophrenia. Proc Natl Acad Sci USA 94:1612–1614, 1997

Barrett S, Beck JC, Bernier R, et al: An autosomal genomic screen for autism: collaborative linkage study of autism. Am J Med Genet 88:609–615, 1999

Bartha R, Williamson PC, Drost DJ, et al: Measurement of glutamate and glutamine in the medial prefrontal cortex of never treated schizophrenic patients and healthy controls by proton magnetic resonance spectroscopy. Arch Gen Psychiatry 54:959–965, 1997

Bassett AS: Chromosomal aberrations and schizophrenia: autosomes. Br J Psychiatry 161:323–334, 1992

Bedwell JS, Keller B, Smith AK, et al: Why does postpsychotic IQ decline in childhood-onset schizophrenia? Am J Psychiatry 156:1996–1997, 1999

Beitchman JH: Childhood schizophrenia: a review and comparison with adult-onset chizophrenia. Psychiatr Clin North Am 8:793–814, 1985

Bertolino A, Kumra S, Callicott JH, et al: Common pattern of cortical pathology in childhood-onset and adult-onset schizophrenia as identified by proton magnetic resonance spectroscopic imaging. Am J Psychiatry 155:1376–1383, 1998

Bilder RM, Goldman RS, Robinson D, et al: Neuropsychology of first-episode schizophrenia: initial characterization and clinical correlates. Am J Psychiatry 157:549–559, 2000

Braff DL, Heaton R, Kuck J, et al: The generalized pattern of neuropsychological deficits in outpatients with chronic schizophrenia with heterogeneous Wisconsin Card Sorting Test results. Arch Gen Psychiatry 48:891–898, 1991

Campbell M, Cueva JE: Psychopharmacology in child and adolescent psychiatry: a review of the past seven years, part I. J Am Acad Child Adolesc Psychiatry 34:1124–1132, 1995a

Campbell M, Cueva JE: Psychopharmacology in child and adolescent psychiatry: a review of the past seven years, part II. J Am Acad Child Adolesc Psychiatry 34:1262–1272, 1995b

Caplan R: Thought disorder in childhood. J Am Acad Child Adolesc Psychiatry 33:605–615, 1994

Chakos MH, Lieberman JA, Alvir J, et al: Caudate nuclei volumes in schizophrenic patients treated with typical antipsychotics or clozapine. Lancet 345:456–457, 1995

Childs B, Scriver CR: Age at onset and causes of disease. Perspect Biol Med 29:437–460, 1986

Chugani HT, Muller RA, Chugani DC: Functional brain reorganization in children. Brain Dev 18:347–356, 1996

Conley RR, Buchanan RW: Evaluation of treatment-resistant schizophrenia. Schizophr Bull 23:663–674, 1997

Cornblatt B, Obuchowski M, Schnur D, et al: Hillside study of risk and early detection in schizophrenia. Br J Psychiatry 172(suppl):26–32, 1998

DeLisi LE, Friedrich U, Wahlstrom J, et al: Schizophrenia and sex chromosome anomalies. Schizophr Bull 20:495–505, 1994

DeLisi LE, Tew W, Xie S, et al: A prospective follow-up study of brain morphology and cognition in first-episode schizophrenic patients: preliminary findings. Biol Psychiatry 38:349–360, 1995

DeLisi LE, Shaw S, Sherrington R, et al: Failure to establish linkage on the X chromosome in 301 families with schizophrenia or schizoaffective disorder. Am J Med Genet 96:335–341, 2000

Egan MF, Goldberg TE, Kolachana BS, et al: Effect of COMT Val108/158 Met genotype on frontal lobe function and risk for schizophrenia. Proc Natl Acad Sci U S A 98:6917–6922, 2001

Eggers C, Bunk D: The long-term course of childhood-onset schizophrenia: a 42-year follow up. Schizophr Bull 23:105–117, 1997

Feinberg I: Schizophrenia: caused by a fault in programmed synaptic elimination during adolescence? J Psychiatr Res 17:319–334, 1982–1983

Folstein SE, Mankoski RE: Chromosome 7q: where autism meets language disorder? Am J Hum Genet 67:278–281, 2000

Folstein S, Rutter M: Genetic influences and infantile autism. Nature 265:726–728, 1997a

Folstein S, Rutter M: Infantile autism: a genetic study of 21 twin pairs. J Child Psychiatry 18:297–321, 1997b

Frazier JA, Giedd JN, Hamburger SD, et al: Brain anatomic magnetic resonance imaging in childhood-onset schizophrenia. Arch Gen Psychiatry 53:617–624, 1996

Frith C: Neuropsychology of schizophrenia: what are the implications of intellectual and experiential abnormalities for the neurobiology of schizophrenia? Br Med Bull 52:618–626, 1996

Galdos PM, Van Os JJ, Murray RM: Puberty and the onset of psychosis. Schizophr Res 10:7–14, 1993

Gershon ES, Badner JA, Goldin LR, et al: Closing in on genes for manic-depressive illness and schizophrenia. Neuropsychopharmacology 18:233–242, 1998

Giedd JN: Neuroimaging of pediatric neuropsychiatric disorders: is a picture really worth a thousand words? Arch Gen Psychiatry 58:443–444, 2001

Giedd JN, Blumenthal J, Jeffries NO, et al: Brain development during childhood and adolescence: a longitudinal MRI study. Nat Neurosci 2:861–863, 1999

Goldberg TE, Gold JM: Neurocognitive functioning in patients with schizophrenia: an overview, in Psychopharmacology: The Fourth Generation of Progress. Edited by Bloom FE, Kupfer DJ. New York, Raven, 1995, pp 1245–1257

Gordon CT, Krasnewich D, White B, et al: Brief report: translocation involving chromosomes 1 and 7 in a boy with childhood-onset schizophrenia. J Autism Dev Disord 24:537–545, 1994a

Gordon CT, Frazier JA, McKenna K, et al: Childhood-onset schizophrenia: an NIMH study in progress. Schizophr Bull 20:697–712, 1994b

Green WH, Padron-Gayol M, Hardesty AS, et al: Schizophrenia with childhood onset: a phenomenological study of 38 cases. J Am Acad Child Adolesc Psychiatry 31:968–976, 1992

Gur RE, Cowell P, Turetsky BI, et al: A follow-up magnetic resonance imaging study of schizophrenia: relationship of neuroanatomical changes to clinical and neurobehavioral measures. Arch Gen Psychiatry 55:145–152, 1998

Hafner H, Nowonty B: Epidemiology of early onset schizophrenia. Eur Arch Psychiatry Clin Neurosci 245:80–92, 1995

Hafner H, Maurer K, Loffler W, et al: The influence of age and sex on the onset and early course of schizophrenia. Br J Psychiatry 162:80–86, 1993

Heaton RK, Gladsjo JA, Palmer BW, et al: Stability and course of neuropsychological deficits in schizophrenia. Arch Gen Psychiatry 58:24–32, 2001

Hollis C: Child and adolescent (juvenile onset) schizophrenia: a case control study of premorbid developmental impairments. Br J Psychiatry 166:489–495, 1995

Hollis C: Adult outcomes of child- and adolescent-onset schizophrenia: diagnostic stability and predictive validity. Am J Psychiatry 157:1652–1659, 2000

Huttenlocher PR: Synaptic density in human frontal cortex-developmental changes and effects of aging. Brain Res 163:195–205, 1979

Jacobsen LK, Rapoport JL: Childhood-onset schizophrenia: implications of clinical and neurobiological research. J Child Psychol Psychiatry 38:697–712, 1998

Jacobsen LK, Hong WL, Hommer DW, et al: Smooth pursuit eye movements in childhood-onset schizophrenia: comparison with attention-deficit hyperactivity disorder and normal controls. Biol Psychiatry 40:1144–1154, 1996a

Jacobsen LK, Giedd JN, Vaituzis AC, et al: Temporal lobe morphology in childhood-onset schizophrenia. Am J Psychiatry 153:355–361, 1996b

Jacobsen LK, Hamburger SD, Van Horn JD, et al: Cerebral glucose metabolism in childhood onset schizophrenia. Psychiatry Res 75:131–144, 1997a

Jacobsen LK, Giedd JN, Rajapakse JC, et al: Quantitative magnetic resonance imaging of the corpus callosum in childhood onset schizophrenia. Psychiatry Res 68:77–86, 1997b

Jacobsen LK, Giedd JN, Berquin PC, et al: Quantitative morphology of the cerebellum and fourth ventricle in childhood-onset schizophrenia. Am J Psychiatry 154:1663–1669, 1997c

Jacobsen LK, Giedd JN, Tanrikut C, et al: Three-dimensional cortical morphometry of the planum temporale in childhood-onset schizophrenia. Am J Psychiatry 154:685–687, 1997d

Jacobsen LK, Giedd JN, Castellanos FX, et al: Progressive reduction of temporal lobe structures in childhood-onset schizophrenia. Am J Psychiatry 155:678–685, 1998

Jones PB, Done J: From birth to onset: a developmental perspective in two national birth cohorts, in Neurodevelopment and Adult Psychopathology. Edited by Keshavan M, Murray RM. New York, Cambridge University Press, 1997, pp 119–136

Kallmann FJ, Roth B: Genetic aspects of preadolescent schizophrenia. Am J Psychiatry 112:599–606, 1956

Karayiorgou M, Gogos JA: A turning point in schizophrenia genetics. Neuron 19:967–979, 1997

Kendler KS: The impact of diagnostic hierarchies on prevalence estimates for psychiatric disorders. Compr Psychiatry 29:218–227, 1988

Kendler KS, Tsuang MT, Hays P: Age at onset in schizophrenia: a familial perspective. Arch Gen Psychiatry 44:881–890, 1987

Kendler KS, McGuire M, Gruenberg AM, et al: The Roscommon Family Study, I: methods, diagnosis of probands, and risk of schizophrenia in relatives. Arch Gen Psychiatry 50:527–540, 1993a

Kendler KS, McGuire M, Gruenberg AM, et al: The Roscommon Family Study, II: the risk of nonschizophrenic nonaffective psychoses in relatives. Arch Gen Psychiatry 50:645–652, 1993b

Kendler KS, McGuire M, Gruenberg AM, et al: The Roscommon Family Study, III: schizophrenia-related personality disorders in relatives. Arch Gen Psychiatry 50:781–788, 1993c

Kendler KS, Gruenberg AM, Kinney DK: Independent diagnoses of adoptees and relatives as defined by DSM-III in the provincial and national samples of the Danish Adoption Study of schizophrenia. Arch Gen Psychiatry 51:456–468, 1994

Kendler KS, Karkowski-Shuman L, Walsh D: Age at onset in schizophrenia and risk of illness in relatives: results from the Roscommon Family Study. Br J Psychiatry 169:213–218, 1996

Kenny JT, Friedman L, Findling RL, et al: Cognitive impairment in adolescents with schizophrenia. Am J Psychiatry 154:1613–1615, 1997

Kernberg PF: Resolved: borderline personality exists in children under twelve. Affirmative. J Am Acad Child Adolesc Psychiatry 29:478–482, 1990

Kolvin I: Studies in the childhood psychoses, I: diagnostic criteria and classification. Br J Psychiatry 118:381–384, 1971

Kremen WS, Faraone SV, Seidman LJ, et al: Neuropsychological risk indicators for schizophrenia: a preliminary study of female relatives of schizophrenic and bipolar probands. Psychiatry Res 79:227–240, 1998

Kumra S, Frazier JA, Jacobsen LK, et al: Childhood-onset schizophrenia: a double-blind clozapine-haloperidol comparison. Arch Gen Psychiatry 53:1090–1097, 1996

Kumra S, Wiggs E, Krasnewich D, et al: Brief report: association of sex chromosome anomalies with childhood-onset psychotic disorders. J Am Acad Child Adolesc Psychiatry 37:292–296, 1998a

Kumra S, Jacobsen LK, Lenane M, et al: Childhood-onset schizophrenia: an open-label study of olanzapine in adolescents. J Am Acad Child Adolesc Psychiatry 37:377–385, 1998b

Kumra S, Jacobsen LK, Lenane M, et al: "Multidimensionally impaired disorder": is it a variant of very early onset schizophrenia? J Am Acad Child Adolesc Psychiatry 37:91–99, 1998c

Kumra S, Giedd JN, Vaituzis AC, et al: Childhood-onset psychotic disorders: magnetic resonance imaging of volumetric differences in brain structure. Am J Psychiatry 157:1467–1474, 2000a

Kumra S, Wiggs E, Bedwell J, et al: Neuropsychological deficits in pediatric patients with childhood-onset schizophrenia and psychotic disorder not otherwise specified. Schizophr Res 42:135–144, 2000b

Kumra S, Sporn A, Hommer D, et al: Smooth pursuit eye tracking impairment in childhood-onset psychotic disorders. Am J Psychiatry, in press

Lai CS, Fisher SE, Hurst JA, et al: The SPCH1 region on human 7q31: genomic characterization of the critical interval and localization of translocations associated with speech and language disorder. Am J Hum Genet 67:357–368, 2000

Levy DL, Holzman PS, Matthysse S, Mendell NR: Eye tracking dysfunction and schizophrenia: a critical perspective. Schizophr Bull 19:461–536 1993

Lieberman JA, Alvir JM, Koreen A, et al: Psychobiologic correlates of treatment response in schizophrenia. Neuropsychopharmacology 14(suppl 3):13-21, 1996

Lim KO, Harris D, Beal M, et al: Gray matter deficits in young onset schizophrenia are independent of age of onset. Biol Psychiatry 40:4–13, 1996

Makowski D, Waternaux C, Lajonchere CM, et al: Thought disorder in adolescent-onset schizophrenia. Schizophr Res 23:147–165, 1997

Marder SR: An approach to treatment resistance in schizophrenia. Br J Psychiatry 37(suppl):19–22, 1999

Marsh L, Harris D, Lim KO, et al: Structural magnetic resonance imaging abnormalities in men with severe chronic schizophrenia and an early age at clinical onset. Arch Gen Psychiatry 54:1104–1112, 1997

Matsumodo H, Simmons A, Williams S, et al: Structural magnetic imaging of the hippocampus in early onset schizophrenia. Biol Psychiatry 49:824–831, 2001

Maziade M, Gingras N, Rodrigue C, et al: Long-term stability of diagnosis and symptom dimensions in a systmatic sample of patients with onset of schizophrenia in childhood and early adolescence, I: nosology, sex and age of onset. Br J Psychiatry 169:361–370, 1996

McClellan J, McCurry C, Snell J, et al: Early-onset psychotic disorders: course and outcome over a 2-year period. J Am Acad Child Adolesc Psychiatry 38:1380–1388, 1999

McKenna K, Gordon CT, Rapoport JL: Childhood-onset schizophrenia: timely neurobiological research. J Am Acad Child Adolesc Psychiatry 33:771–781, 1994a

McKenna K, Gordon CT, Lenane M, et al: Looking for childhood-onset schizophrenia: the first 71 cases screened. J Am Acad Child Adolesc Psychiatry 33:636–644, 1994b

Moore GJ, Bebchuk JM, Wilds IB, et al: Lithium-induced increase in human brain gray matter. Lancet 356:1241–1242, 2000

Mors O, Mortensen PB, Ewald H: No evidence of increased risk for schizophrenia or bipolar affective disorder in persons with aneuploidies of the sex chromosomes. Psychol Med 31:425–430, 2001

Nelson MD, Saykin AJ, Flashman LA, et al: Hippocampal volume reduction in schizophrenia as assessed by magnetic resonance imaging: a meta-analytic study. Arch Gen Psychiatry 433–440, 1998

Nopoulos PC, Giedd JN, Andreasen NC, et al: Frequency and severity of enlarged cavum septi pellucidi in childhood-onset schizophrenia. Am J Psychiatry 155:1074–1079, 1998

Orvaschel H, Tabrizi MA, Chambers W: Schedule for Affective Disorders and Schizophrenia for School-Age Children: Epidemiologic Version, 3rd Edition. New York, New York State Psychiatric Institute and Yale University School of Medicine, 1980

Parnas J, Schulsinger F, Schulsinger H, et al: Behavioral precursors of schizophrenia spectrum: a prospective study. Arch Gen Psychiatry 39:658–664, 1982

Paterson AD: Sixth World Congress of Psychiatric Genetics X Chromosome Workshop. Am J Med Genet 88:279–286, 1999

Paulsen JS, Heaton RK, Sadek JR, et al: The nature of learning and memory impairments in schizophrenia. J Int Neuropsychol Soc 1:88–99, 1995

Pickar D, Owen RR, Litman RE, et al: Clinical and biologic response to clozapine in patients with schizophrenia: crossover comparison with fluphenazine. Arch Gen Psychiatry 49:345–353, 1992

Pool D, Bloom W, Mielke DH, et al: A controlled evaluation of loxitane in seventy-five adolescent schizophrenic patients. Curr Ther Res Clin Exp 19:99–104, 1976

Poulton R, Caspi A, Moffitt TE, et al: Children's self-reported psychotic symptoms and adult schizophreniform disorder: a 15-year longitudinal study. Arch Gen Psychiatry 57:1053–1058, 2000

Rapoport JL, Inoff-Germain G: Update on childhood-onset schizophrenia. Curr Psychiatry Rep 2:410–415, 2000

Rapoport JL, Giedd J, Kumra S, et al: Childhood-onset schizophrenia: progressive ventricular change during adolescence. Arch Gen Psychiatry 54:897–903, 1997

Rapoport JL, Giedd JN, Blumenthal J, et al: Progressive cortical change during adolescence in childhood-onset schizophrenia: a longitudinal magnetic resonance imaging study. Arch Gen Psychiatry 56:649–654, 1999

Russell AT: The clinical presentation of childhood-onset schizophrenia. Schizophr Bull 20:631–646, 1994

Saykin AJ, Shtasel DL, Gur RE, et al: Neuropsychological deficits in neuroleptic naïve patients with first-episode schizophrenia. Arch Gen Psychiatry 51:124–131, 1994

Schmidt M, Blanz B, Dippe A, et al: Course of patients diagnosed as having schizophrenia during first episode occurring under age 18 years. Eur Arch Psychiatry Clin Neurosci 245:93–100, 1995

Selemon LD, Goldman-Rakic PS: The reduced neuropil hypothesis: a circuit-based model of schizophrenia. Biol Psychiatry 45:17–25, 1999

Shenton ME, Wible CG, McCarley RW: A review of magnetic resonance imaging studies of brain abnormalities in schizophrenia, in Brain Imaging in Clinical Psychiatry. Edited by Krishnan KRR, Doraiswamy PM. New York, Marcel Dekker, 1997, pp 297–380

Sowell ER, Levitt J, Thompson PM, et al: Brain abnormalities in early-onset schizophrenia spectrum disorder observed with statistical parametric mapping of structural magnetic resonance images. Am J Psychiatry 157:1475–1484, 2000

Spencer EK, Campbell M: Children with schizophrenia: diagnosis, phenomenology, and pharmacotherapy. Schizophr Bull 20:713–725, 1994

Spencer EK, Kafantaris V, Padron-Gayol MV, et al: Haloperidol in schizophrenic children: early findings from a study in progress. Psychopharmacol Bull 28:183–186, 1992

Toniolo D, D'Adamo P: X-linked nonspecific mental retardation. Curr Opin Genet Dev 10:280–285, 2000

Towbin KE, Dykens EM, Pearson GS, et al: Conceptualizing "borderline syndrome of childhood" and "childhood schizophrenia" as a developmental disorder. J Am Acad Child Adolesc Psychiatry 32:775–782, 1993

Tsuang MT, Stone WS, Faraone SVL: Genes, environment and schizophrenia. Br J Psychiatry 40(suppl):S18–S24, 2001

Turetz M, Mozes T, Toren P, et al: An open trial of clozapine in neuroleptic-resistant childhood-onset schizophrenia. Br J Psychiatry 170:507–510, 1997

Usiskin SI, Nicolson R, Krasnewich DM, et al: Velocardiofacial syndrome in childhood-onset schizophrenia. J Am Acad Child Adolesc Psychiatry 38:1536–1543, 1999

Walker EF, Savoie T, Davis D: Neuromotor precursors of schizophrenia. Schizophr Bull 20:441–451, 1994

Warburton P, Baird G, Chen W, et al: Support for linkage of autism and specific language impairment to 7q3 from two chromosome rearrangements involving band 7q31. Am J Med Genet 96:228–234, 2000

Watkins JM, Asarnow RF, Tanguay PE: Symptom development in childhood onset schizophrenia. J Child Psychol Psychiatry 29:865–878, 1988

Werry JS: Childhood schizophrenia, in Psychoses and Pervasive Developmental Disorders in Childhood and Adolescence. Edited by Volkmar FR. Washington, DC, American Psychiatric Press, 1996, pp 1–48

Werry JS, McClellan JM: Predicting outcome in child and adolescent (early onset) schizophrenia and bipolar disorder. J Am Acad Child Adolesc Psychiatry 31:147–150, 1992

Werry JS, McClellan JM, Chard L: Childhood and adolescent schizophrenic, bipolar, and schizoaffective disorders: a clinical and outcome study. J Am Acad Child Adolesc Psychiatry 30:457–465, 1991

Zahn TP, Jacobsen LK, Gordon CT, et al: Autonomic nervous system markers of psychopathology in childhood-onset schizophrenia. Arch Gen Psychiatry 54:904–912, 1997

8

Schizophrenia During Adolescence

S. Charles Schulz, M.D.

Robert L. Findling, M.D.

Marilyn A. Davies, Ph.D.

Schizophrenia is a severe and debilitating psychiatric disease that afflicts 1% of the world's population. The average age at onset of this psychotic disorder is estimated to be between 19 and 23 years of age (Hafner et al. 1993; Loranger 1984), with males having an earlier age at onset. Interestingly, Loranger's study demonstrates that as many as 39% of males with schizophrenia had their first psychotic episode before age 19. The etiology of schizophrenia remains unknown, but there is strong epidemiologic evidence for a genetic vulnerability. During the past decade, a neurodevelopmental model of schizophrenia has been widely discussed as a means of understanding results of brain imaging and neuropsychological test results (Weinberger 1987). Bolstering a neurodevelopmental hypothesis for the pathophysiology of schizophrenia are recent studies indicating that patients who later become schizophrenic have different responses to psychological and motoric examinations many years before the onset of psychotic symptoms (as early as 6 years old) (Jones et al. 1994). Given this backdrop, one may question why there would be a specific focus on schizophrenia occurring in adolescents. There are actually a number of important reasons for attention to schizophrenia in this younger age group:

1. Adolescence represents an important phase of central nervous system development; therefore, etiologically important clues may be gained from neuropsychiatric studies.
2. New pharmacologic interventions have become available that have been shown to be more effective and safer in adults with schizophrenia. These new treatments may lead to programs for early intervention, as described in Chapter 1, and for early detection of psychosis in adolescents.
3. Despite the opinion of numerous investigators that schizophrenia in adolescents is part of the continuum of the adult illness, psychosocial treatments, especially family treatments, may need to be tailored for these patients and their families. Significant psychological events unfold during the teenage years, which are probably altered by or interact with the prodrome or onset of schizophrenia, requiring specific clinical programs.
4. A review of the literature indicates that the adolescent stage of schizophrenia is understudied from the vantage point of empirical research. This may be a result of the division of child and adolescent services from adult care sites.

The purpose of this chapter is to describe the known epidemiology of schizophrenia in teenagers, review recent brain imaging research in adolescent schizophrenic patients, review studies of the pharmacologic approach to these patients, and describe our emerging data that may point to specific family approaches.

Epidemiology

Although the epidemiology of schizophrenia has been well studied, little direct information exists on the epidemiology of schizophrenia before age 18. We can glean some information from first-admission studies that have investigated the age at onset of psychotic illnesses.

Loranger (1984) examined first-admission patients to determine the age at onset and age of first treatment to study whether males had an earlier age at onset of schizophrenia than females. An analysis of the results of his study indicates that whereas 39% of males had onset of schizophrenia before age 19 years, 23% of females had experienced their first psychotic symptoms by that age. An examination of these results would indicate that adolescent onset of schizophrenia is not a rare event, because a substantial proportion of males and females experience the illness for the first time before reaching age 20 years. Also, Loranger (1984) concluded that there was evidence for earlier onset in males, a finding that may influence the design of services for the adolescent group of patients.

Hafner et al. (1993) also used the examination of a first-treatment group to explore age at onset and potential differences between males and females and confirmed Loranger's earlier findings of earlier male onset. In their studies, males had an approximate 4-year earlier onset of prodrome, first symptoms, and first treatment. Hafner's findings were not identical to Loranger's, however, in that the average age at onset of psychotic symptoms was later. Therefore, we conclude that many patients have the beginning of schizophrenia in adolescence, but few studies or descriptions exist of these young patients' characteristics or treatment.

The earlier onset of schizophrenia in males is a tantalizing clue to the etiology of schizophrenia. Based on the later onset in females through adolescence and young adulthood, investigators have hypothesized a protective effect of estrogen (Galdos et al. 1993). MRI studies to date indicate that males with schizophrenia may differ more than females with schizophrenia from healthy control subjects, thus suggesting that there might be pathophysiological differences (Nopolous et al. 1997). However, not all studies have confirmed this finding. Further studies in teenagers, perhaps involving careful staging of puberty in both genders, may contribute to this line of research.

In an important epidemiologic assessment of first-admission psychotic patients, Bromet et al. (1992) assessed all first-admission psychotic patients to Suffolk County Hospitals, Long Island, New York (see Chapter 2). Of note in this study is the finding that when the diagnosis of schizophrenia was made at the index admission, it was highly stable over the next 6 months to a statistically significant degree (Carlson et. al 1994). This is a crucial finding for the biology and pharmacology sections that follow because it supports the idea that young people given the diagnosis of schizophrenia retain the diagnosis over a substantial period of time.

Therefore, epidemiologic surveys of first-episode patients indicate that onset of symptoms in the teenage years is not a rare event and that familiarity with schizophrenia in this age group is important for clinicians and investigators. However, it must be noted that our understanding of fundamental epidemiological questions regarding adolescents remains scant. For example, we do not know with certainty whether adolescent schizophrenia is a more severe form of the disorder because of its earlier onset or whether adolescents with schizophrenia may have a longer prodrome and a more insidious onset. Furthermore, assessment of gender differences in young patients has only just begun. Clearly, further attention to these important details is needed, a need that can probably be answered only by prospective studies of adolescent patients.

Brain Imaging Studies

The development of computer-assisted tomography (CAT) scanning techniques ushered in a new era of psychiatric research, especially for seriously psychiatrically ill patients. Early examinations of CAT scans did not reveal a pathognomonic lesion in patients suffering from schizophrenia, so it was not until Johnstone et al. (1976) first used quantitation of ventricular size in CAT scans that differences between schizophrenic patients and control subjects were found.

Subsequent studies by Weinberger et al. (1979) confirmed the existence of enlarged ventricles in schizophrenic patients as compared with control subjects. Since then, numerous studies have been performed showing that enlarged ventricles are statistically significantly seen in schizophrenic patients (see meta-analyses by Raz and Raz [1990] and Elkis et al. [1995]). Despite the numerous computed tomography (CT) and magnetic resonance imaging (MRI) studies of patients with schizophrenia, very little work was done in younger patients. Weinberger et al. (1982) showed that schizophreniform patients had enlarged ventricles just as did chronic patients. These early CAT scan studies were later extended to first-episode MRI studies by DeLisi et al. (1991) and Degreef et al. (1992). Both first-episode reports studied patients of a mean age in the midtwenties and showed that there were substantial increases in ventricular size as well as temporal lobe abnormalities. These studies of schizophreniform or first-episode patients demonstrating brain imaging abnormalities at the outset of the illness are key contributions to the neurodevelopmental hypothesis of schizophrenia. However, because first-episode studies are almost always performed on adult inpatient units, few studies have been performed on adolescent patients with schizophrenia.

In the early 1980s, Schulz et al. (1983) assessed ventricular size in teenagers with schizophrenia and in teenagers who were without psychosis but had borderline personality disorder. They were compared with similarly aged medical record control subjects. The teenagers with schizophrenia (mean age, 16 years) had enlarged ventricles compared with both comparison groups. Further studies indicated an association between ventricular size and treatment response (Schulz et al. 1983) and a statistical relationship of ventricular size with monoamine metabolites in the cerebrospinal fluid (CSF; Jennings et al. 1985). At the same time, other groups noted ventricular enlargement in case series (Findling et al. 1995). Such studies demonstrated that ventriculomegaly could occur much earlier than had been reported previously (Weinberger et al. 1982). The adolescent studies further bolstered a neurodevelopmental hypothesis of schizophrenia and underscored the continuity (at least as assessed by brain imaging) between the pathophysiology in adolescent and in adult patients.

Since the advent of MRI scanning, another attempt has been made to explore schizophrenia in adolescents. MRI clearly allows for a more refined anatomic assessment and the ability to make volumetric measures of general brain parameters (i.e., ventricular size) and of specific brain structures such as the thalamus and hippocampus.

Using MRI, Frazier et al. (1996) assessed a group of adolescents with childhood-onset schizophrenia (COS) versus control subjects and demonstrated a smaller brain size, smaller thalamus, and nearly significantly enlarged ventricular size (see Chapter 7). Interestingly, this same research group recently reported a 2-year follow-up study that indicated that ventricular size enlarged in adolescents with COS compared with age-matched controls (Rapoport et al. 1997). This latter finding does not refute the neurodevelopmental theory of schizophrenia, but it does add an interesting dimension to studies using MRI. As indicated earlier, adolescence is a particularly active time in brain development, and the findings by Rapoport et al. (1997) of ventricular enlargement over time may indicate an interaction of neurodevelopment with disease-related progression of brain changes.

Our research group has been studying adolescents with schizophrenia and bipolar illness and control subjects and has observed results similar to those reported by Frazier et al. (1996). In contrast to the National Institute of Mental Health (NIMH) group's studies (Frazier et al. 1996), our patient population is not of childhood onset (with some exceptions) and has an added feature: a comparative group of adolescents with bipolar disorder. Specifically, Friedman et al. (1999) reported that adolescent schizophrenic and bipolar patients have decreased brain volume and increased percentages of CSF in the frontal cortical and temporal cortical areas. These results of general brain measures are complementary to those for the adolescent patients with COS studied by Frazier et al. (1996). Recalling the issue of specificity, the results extend previous studies by demonstrating that adolescents with bipolar disorder also have reduced brain size and increased CSF percentages in the frontal and temporal areas.

Recently, Dasari et al. (1999) analyzed the Friedman et al. (1999) data cited above and found decreased thalamic area in the adolescent patients with schizophrenia. These findings again complement the childhood-onset sample (Frazier et al. 1996).

Brain structure is only one aspect of brain study, so it is interesting that Lys et al. (1999) reported that adolescents with schizophrenia also have MRI spectroscopy differences from control subjects and autistic adolescents. In this study, autistic adolescents were chosen as a comparison group because of the clear neurodevelopmental nature of that illness. The report of decreased N-acetyl-aspartate (NAA) in teenage patients with schizophrenia is consistent with reports by Lim et al. (1998) and indicates that there may be decreased neuronal mass in the frontal area of interest. Of further interest was the similarly decreased NAA in the autistic group.

In summary, studies of adolescent patients with schizophrenia demonstrate structural and functional differences from control subjects in directions and degrees that are similar to those observed in adult patients. In the one follow-up study of adolescents with schizophrenia, Rapoport et al. (1997) have reported a progressive increase over time in ventricular volume in adolescent patients with COS compared with control subjects, thus pointing to possible importance of imaging studies for studying the possibility of progressive brain change during this important stage of brain development.

Furthermore, the biological continuity between adolescent and adult schizophrenia argues for the importance of early intervention with pharmacologic treatment. First, evidence suggests that the longer schizophrenia goes untreated, the poorer the outcome. Second, it follows that teenagers with schizophrenia should be treated as early as possible to enhance a positive course.

Pharmacological Treatment

As previously noted, very few medication studies exist for patients with schizophrenia who are younger than age 18. In the only placebo-controlled study, Pool et al. (1976) noted that haloperidol and loxapine were superior to placebo. They noted a reduction in positive symptoms, thus providing empiric evidence for antipsychotic activity. Although the traditional antipsychotic medications had long been known to be efficacious in adults, not every medication that works in adults has equal effect in adolescents. For example, it has not been possible to demonstrate that tricyclic antidepressant agents are effective in this age group. In the only other controlled trial with traditional antipsychotic medications, Realmuto et al. (1984) noted that thioridazine was equivalent to thiothixene as assessed with objective measures of psychopathology. Although antipsychotic medications reduced symptoms of psychosis, they noted a substantial problem: many patients were neuroleptic intolerant. Therefore, the few available studies of antipsychotic medication in teenagers suggest that the medications are efficacious but poorly tolerated.

Despite the efficacy of the antipsychotic medications in teenagers, there has been substantial reluctance to use the medications because of movement disorder side effects (i.e., dystonia, parkinsonism, and akathisia). Also, antipsychotic medications have been somewhat reluctantly used because of concerns about tardive dyskinesia in a group of patients who may require prolonged periods of treatment.

With the advent of front-line atypical antipsychotic medications came the opportunity to explore whether these new agents were efficacious, safe, and well tolerated in an adolescent population.

As with many new treatments, the first reports were small case studies that indicated that risperidone was an effective and well-tolerated antipsychotic medication in schizophrenic youth (Quintana and Keshavan 1995). Simeon et al. (1995) also reported that risperidone was useful for schizophrenic youngsters as well as youngsters suffering from other psychotic disorders. Although such reports were encouraging, Mandoki (1995) indicated that there might be substantial side effects when risperidone was used in young people.

These findings led our group to explore the use of risperidone in adolescents suffering from schizophrenia. We described a group of 16 adolescents with a mean age of 15 years who received risperidone in average dosages of 6 mg/day and found that positive as well as negative symptoms were statistically reduced. In addition, Clinical Global Impressions (CGI) assessments showed improvement. The study was started shortly after risperidone was released, which explains the relatively high dosages reported. Just as the average dosage of risperidone has gone down in recent years, so has the dosage we use in adolescents. It needs to be pointed out that this study was not placebo controlled and that risperidone was not compared with another antipsychotic medication. Nonetheless, the results are encouraging (Grcevich et al. 1996).

Olanzapine was the second front-line atypical antipsychotic agent to be approved in the United States. Our group is currently examining the efficacy of and appropriate dosing strategy for this compound. We reported the results of the first six patients to complete an open-label, objective rating protocol at the recent International Congress on Schizophrenia Research. Five of the six patients had substantial improvement in CGI rating as well as reduction in Positive and Negative Syndrome Scale for Schizophrenia (PANSS) ratings. The average dosage for adolescents in this study was 15 mg/day. The medication was well tolerated and did not lead to movement disorder side effects (Schulz et al. 1999). Kumra et al. (1998) have also examined the use of olanzapine in adolescents with COS who were previously not responsive to traditional medications. As described in Chapter 7, olanzapine is useful but not as effective as clozapine in this group.

Reflecting on the reports of pharmacotherapy to date, we feel that the new atypical antipsychotic medications should be prescribed because tolerability is critical and the new medications are well accepted by adolescents with schizophrenia. Since our initial report on risperidone use in adolescents, we have began using a lower starting dosage (1–2 mg/day) and slower titration. Our clinical experience with olanzapine has found it to be a safe and useful agent, yet a specific dosing strategy has not emerged.

The medication quetiapine has been reported to successfully reduce symptoms of psychosis in a group of psychotic adolescents (McConville et al. 2000). This group included a majority of patients with bipolar disorder, yet one can clearly consider the role for quetiapine in adolescents with a psychotic illness. Recently, Szigethy et al. (1998) described a case of schizophrenia in adolescence in which neither risperidone nor olanzapine led to lasting relief of symptoms. Subsequently, there was a response to quetiapine at 200 mg/day. They noted that perhaps not all of the new agents are equivalent and that there may be a role for quetiapine in those who have not responded well to other agents.

In summary, the data addressing antipsychotic medications for treating adolescent patients with schizophrenia is scanty, yet case series with the new agents reveal symptom reduction with few movement disorder side effects. In our experience with traditional antipsychotic medications, side effects were very disruptive at the initiation of treatment, an issue that is reduced with the atypical medications. Although our work and that of others show symptom reduction and safety, it is clear that the best dosing strategies for these young patients have yet to be determined. Also, movement disorder side effects are low, but other side effects such as galactorrhea and weight gain require further evaluation.

A Family Perspective

As our work with adolescents progressed, we became increasingly concerned about the families of our young patients. Many family members told us of their needs for support and related the difficulties they had encountered. We noticed they were younger than the parents of our other patients and were in contact with the mental health system for the first time. We now turn to our thoughts about this important issue.

More than three decades of research indicates that families who live with persons with a serious mental illness and take responsibility for their welfare experience difficulties as they try to adjust to the disruption in their lives (Creer and Wing 1975; Doll 1976; Hoenig and Hamilton 1969; Kint 1977; Noh and Turner 1987; Solomon and Draine 1995). These difficulties may take the form of psychological distress, social disruptions, physical illness, or economic hardship. Because the family is undisputed as the primary caregiving system for adolescents with serious mental illness, family members usually suffer considerable burden in coping with the patient's psychiatric illness.

In our study (Davies et al. 1997), which examined the burden of 52 primary caregivers (defined as the person who assumed the major responsibility for the care of the severely mentally ill adolescent), we found that caregivers (mostly parents) reported moderate levels of subjective burden, specifically related to certain adolescent behaviors and one area of social performance. Regarding adolescent behaviors, four were moderately distressing: worry, forgetfulness, misery, and indecisiveness. Not surprising, although reported in only 25% of the adolescents, the most severe levels of subjective caregiver burden were related to the behaviors of violence (i.e., threatening or abuse toward the informant or anyone else) and parasuicide (i.e., adolescent's speaking about taking his or her life). Regarding social performance, caregivers were most distressed about their adolescent's work and study performance. During our semistructured interviews, many parents shared their concerns about inflexible school systems and unknowledgeable teachers. In addition, they shared worries about future academic and schooling issues.

In our opinion, after reflecting on our work with families, most caregivers need many services, including 1) psychoeducation about the nature of the mental illness and normal adolescent behavior and problems; 2) practical advice about what to expect over the course of the mental illness; 3) respite time for psychological distance from the child or adolescent; 4) crisis management support; and 5) referrals to specialized programs and agencies.

Research indicates that support groups are the most efficacious and cost-effective medium for practical advice. Support groups also reduce caregivers' social isolation and allow exposure to the first-hand experience of other parents and caregivers. They are also informational regarding community resources and avoid the stigma of a formal therapeutic setting run by professionals (Budd and Hughes 1997). Although psychoeducation or peer support can both reduce perceptions of burden related to prevalent patient behaviors (e.g., worry and indecisiveness) and social performance issues (e.g., school and study), crisis management support should be available for highly distressing behaviors such as violence and suicidal behaviors. In contrast, distressed caregivers and parents have need of more specialized services that include cognitive therapy. Individual family interventions can help when caregivers demonstrate rigid or fixed blaming attributions or have severe depression or anxiety.

Not all families with a dysfunctional child are dysfunctional. Previous studies indicate that 50%–70% of families with a severely mentally ill child report some problem areas (compared with 30%–50% of normal families). In our study, we determined that no profiles or dimension clusters successfully distinguished functional from dysfunctional families; rather, each family had its unique pattern of function. Generally, most families could benefit from psychoeducation sessions, which provide information related to the illness, its usual course, the monitoring of emerging patient behaviors, problem solving, and skill building (e.g., communication and behavior management).

Perhaps the most prominent data in schizophrenia research relates to the effects of the household or family environment on patient outcome. Although it is well established that patients who live with relatives who are highly critical or emotionally overinvolved (i.e., have high expressed emotion) have a higher probability of relapse than patients who do not show high expressed emotion attitudes (Berkowitz et al. 1984; Brown et al. 1972; Kreisman et al. 1979; Vaughn and Leff 1976; Vaughn et al. 1984), few studies have examined these environmental effects in families of adolescents. However, many family treatment programs include either educational or supportive interventions directed at reducing high expressed emotion, improving family attitudes (Faloon and Peterson 1985; Haas et al. 1988), or improving family function (Abramowitz and Coursey 1989; Faloon and Peterson 1985). Predictably, new patient behaviors and social problems arise that require crisis management or additional professional support. In contrast, our experience indicates that more dysfunctional families need family therapy. We believe this is an important factor in treatment planning—that not all families need the same amount or type of treatment. Those with the greatest problems need more attention at this time.

Lastly, a longitudinal perspective should be considered because families are in varying phases of their normal life-cycle experiences and varying phases of responding to the child's or adolescent's mental illness. For example, although many families need assistance with normal problems, such as setting limits and defining boundaries between parents and children, they are also struggling with feelings about the mental illness that range from shock and disbelief to pessimism about the future. Our sample demonstrated a wide variation in the length of time that families were struggling with the adolescent's psychiatric disorder. Although approximately 25% of our families were relatively early in the process of dealing with the psychiatric illness (<1 year), 20% had been dealing with it for more than 5 years. The duration of the illness was statistically related to the family's level of optimism; longer-term families tended to be pessimistic about their adolescent's future. We believe family members may be more willing to participate if services are designed to meet their specific needs.

Conclusions

This chapter describes a group of studies related to schizophrenia in adolescents. We believe that these studies are important for both clinicians and investigators because of the paucity of data collected on schizophrenic patients while they are teenagers and the lack of clinical trials in this age group. Because adolescents with schizophrenia are traversing important phases in brain and psychological development, it is important that their clinical management reflect their unique needs.

References

Abramowitz IR, Coursey RD: Impact of an educational group on family participants who take care of their schizophrenic relatives. J Consult Clin Psychol 57:232–236, 1989

Berkowitz R, Eberlum-Fries R, Kulpers L, et al: Educating relatives about schizophrenia. Schizophr Bull 10:418–429, 1984

Bromet EJ, Schwartz JE, Fennig S, et al: The epidemiology of psychosis: the Suffolk County Mental Health Project. Schizophr Bull 18:243–255, 1992

Brown GW, Birley JLT, Wing JK: Influence of family life on the course of schizophrenic disorders: a replication. Br J Psychiatry 121:241–258, 1972

Budd RJ, Hughes IC: What do relatives of people with schizophrenia find helpful about family intervention? Schizophr Bull 23:341–347, 1997

Carlson GA, Fennig SD, Bromet E: The confusion between bipolar disorder and schizophrenia in youth: where does it stand in the 1990s? J Am Acad Child Adolesc Psychiatry 33:453–460, 1994

Creer C, Wing J: Living with a schizophrenic patient. Br J Hosp Med July:73–82, 1975

Dasari M, Friedman L, Jesberger JA, et al: A magnetic resonance imaging study of thalamic area in adolescent patients with either schizophrenia or bipolar disorder as compared to healthy controls. Psychiatry Res 91:155–162, 1999

Davies MA, Schulz SC, Meltzer HY, et al: Needs of families and caregivers of psychotic adolescents. Paper presented at American Psychiatric Association Annual Meeting, San Diego, CA, May, 1997

Degreef G, Ashtari M, Bogerts B, et al: Volumes of ventricular system subdivisions measured from magnetic resonance images in first-episode schizophrenic patients. Arch Gen Psychiatry 49:531–537, 1992

DeLisi LE, Hoff AL, Schwartz JE, et al: Brain morphology in first-episode schizophrenic-like psychotic patients: a quantitative magnetic resonance imaging study. Biol Psychiatry 29:159–175, 1991

Doll W: Family coping with the mentally ill: an unanticipated consequence of deinstitutionalization. Hospital and Community Psychiatry 27:183–185, 1976

Elkis H, Friedman L, Wise A, et al: Meta-analyses of studies of ventricular enlargement and cortical sulcal prominence in mood disorders: comparison with controls or patients with schizophrenia. Arch Gen Psychiatry 52:735–746, 1995

Faloon IRH, Peterson J: Family management in the prevention of morbidity of schizophrenia: the adjustment of the family unit. Br J Psychiatry 147:156–163, 1985

Findling RL, Friedman L, Kenny JT, et al: Adolescent schizophrenia: a methodologic review of the current neuroimaging and neuropsychologic literature. J Autism Dev Disord 25:627–639, 1995

Friedman L, Findling RL, Kenny JT, et al: A magnetic resonance imaging study of adolescent patients with either schizophrenia or bipolar disorder as compared to healthy controls. Biol Psychiatry 46:78–88, 1999

Frazier JA, Giedd JN, Hamburger SD, et al: Brain anatomic magnetic resonance imaging in childhood-onset schizophrenia. Arch Gen Psychiatry 53:617–624, 1996

Galdos PM, van Os JJ, Murray RM: Puberty and the onset of psychosis. Schizophr Res 10:7–14, 1993

Grcevich SJ, Findling RL, Rowane WA, et al: Risperidone in the treatment of children and adolescents with schizophrenia: a retrospective study. J Child Adol Psychopharmacol 6:251–257, 1996

Haas GL, Glick ID, Clarkin JF, et al: Inpatient family intervention: a randomized clinical trial. Arch Gen Psychiatry 45:217–224, 1988

Hafner H, Maurer K, Loffler W, et al: The influence of age and sex on the onset and early course of schizophrenia. Br J Psychiatry 162:80–86, 1993

Hoenig J, Hamilton MW: The Desegregation of the Mentally Ill. London, Routledge, 1969

Jennings WS Jr, Schulz SC, Narasimhachari N, et al: Brain ventricular size and CSF monoamine metabolites in an adolescent inpatient population. Psychiatry Res 16:87–94 1985

Johnstone EC, Crow TJ, Frith CD, et al: Cerebral ventricular size and cognitive impairment in chronic schizophrenia. Lancet 2:924–926, 1976

Jones P, Rodgers B, Murray R, et al: Child developmental risk factors for adult schizophrenia in the British 1946 birth cohort. Lancet 344:1398–1402, 1994

Kint MG: Problems for families vs. problem families. Schizophr Bull 3:355–356, 1977

Kreisman DE, Simmens SJ, Joy VD: Rejecting the patient: preliminary validation of a self-report scale. Schizophr Bull 5:220–223, 1979

Kumra S, Jacobsen LK, Lenane M, et al: Childhood-onset schizophrenia: an open-label study of olanzapine in adolescents. J Am Acad Child Adolesc Psychiatry 37:377–385, 1998

Lim KO, Adalsteinsson E, Spielman D, et al: Proton magnetic resonance spectroscopic imaging of cortical gray and white matter in schizophrenia. Arch Gen Psychiatry 55:346–352, 1998

Loranger AW: Sex differences in age of onset of schizophrenia. Arch Gen Psychiatry 41:157–161, 1984

Lys C, Findling L, Friedman S, et al: Frontal lobe metabolism and aberrant neurodevelopment: a comparative MRS study among adolescents with autism, schizophrenia and healthy subjects. Schizophr Res 36:226, 1999

Mandoki MW: Risperidone treatment of children and adolescents: increased risk of extrapyramidal side effects? J Child Adolesc Psychopharmacol 5:49–67, 1995

McConville BJ, Arvantis LA, Thyrum PT, et al: Pharmacokinetics, tolerability, and clinical effectiveness of quetiapine fumarate: an open-label trial in adolescents with psychotic disorders. J Clin Psychiatry 61:252–260, 2000

Noh S, Turner RJ: Living with psychiatric patients: implications for the mental health of family members. Soc Sci Med 25:263–271, 1987

Nopoulos P, Flaum M, Andreasen NC: Sex differences in brain morphology in schizophrenia. Am J Psychiatry 154:1637–1639, 1997

Pool D, Bloom W, Mielke DH, et al: A controlled evaluation of Loxitane in seventy-five adolescent schizophrenic patients. Curr Ther Res Clin Exp 19:99–104, 1976

Quintana H, Keshavan M: Risperidone in children and adolescents with schizophrenia. J Am Acad Child Adolesc Psychiatry 34:1292–1296, 1995

Rapoport JL, Giedd J, Kumra S, et al: Childhood-onset schizophrenia: progressive ventricular change during adolescence. Arch Gen Psychiatry 54:897–903, 1997

Raz S, Raz N: Structural brain abnormalities in the major psychoses: a quantitative review of the evidence from computerized imaging. Psychol Bull 108:93–108, 1990

Realmuto GM, Erickson WD, Yellin AM, et al: Clinical comparison of thiothixene and thioridazine in schizophrenic adolescents. Am J Psychiatry 141:440–442, 1984

Schulz SC, Koller MM, Kishore PR, et al: Ventricular enlargements in teenage patients with schizophrenia spectrum disorder. Am J Psychiatry 140:1592–1595, 1983

Schulz SC, Findling RL, Branicky LA, et al: Olanzapine in adolescents with a psychotic disorder. Schizophr Res 36:297, 1999

Simeon JG, Carrey NJ, Wiggins DM, et al: Risperidone effects in treatment-resistant adolescents: preliminary case reports. J Child Adolesc Psychopharmacol 5:69–79, 1995

Solomon P, Draine J: Adaptive coping among family members of persons with serious mental illness. Psychiatr Serv 46:1156–1160, 1995

Szigethy E, Brent S, Findling R: Quetiapine for refractory schizophrenia. J Am Acad Child Adolesc Psychiatry 37:1127–1128, 1998

Vaughn CE, Leff JP: The influence of family and social factors on the outcome of psychiatric illness: a comparison of schizophrenic and depressed neurotic patients. Br J Psychiatry 129:125–137, 1976

Vaughn CE, Snyder KS, Jones S, et al: Family factors in schizophrenic relapse: replication in California of British research on expressed emotion. Arch Gen Psychiatry 41:1169–1177, 1984

Weinberger DR: Implications of normal brain development in the pathogenesis of schizophrenia. Arch Gen Psychiatry 44:660–669, 1987

Weinberger DR, Torrey EF, Neophytides AN, et al: Lateral cerebral ventricular enlargement in chronic schizophrenia. Arch Gen Psychiatry 36:735–739, 1979

Weinberger DR, DeLisis LE, Perman GP, et al: Computed tomography in schizophreniform disorder and other acute psychiatric disorders. Arch Gen Psychiatry 39:778–783, 1982

9

Cognitive Impairment in Early-Stage Schizophrenia

John T. Kenny, Ph.D.

Lee Friedman, Ph.D.

This chapter begins with an overview of cognitive deficits in adult schizophrenia. The purpose is to provide a broader developmental framework, because the issue of whether schizophrenia has a neurodevelopmental or neurodegenerative etiology has been paramount (Murray et al. 1988; Weinberger 1987). Although both imply a neurobiological etiology, the distinction between them is the point along the developmental trajectory at which the cognitive disruption is presumed to have occurred. The psychopathological specificity of cognitive dysfunction is also addressed, in terms of both diagnosis and symptom presentation (i.e., psychosis versus nonpsychosis and negative versus positive symptoms), as is the functional outcome of neurocognitive dysfunction. The pharmacologic and cognitive rehabilitative aspects of neuropsychological dysfunction in schizophrenia are also briefly reviewed.

We then discuss issues related to cognitive deficits in early-stage schizophrenia (e.g., first-episode adult schizophrenia, adolescent-onset versus adult-onset schizophrenia, adolescents with schizophrenia, children with schizophrenia, and pre- versus postpsychotic cognitive functioning in schizophrenia). For the purpose of discussion, "early-stage schizophrenia" can refer to either the stage of chronological development or the stage of illness onset.

The chapter focuses primarily on studies that have used clinical cognitive measures rather than experimental procedures (i.e., reaction time, span of apprehension).

Cognitive Deficits in Adult Schizophrenia

Identified cognitive deficits in adult patients with schizophrenia affect attention, memory, and executive functions involving problem solving, planning, and organization. A recent meta-analysis encompassing a large sample of patients showed that any selectivity of a specific cognitive deficit in schizophrenia is relatively mild and occurs in the context of a much broader-based global impairment in cognition (Heinrichs and Zakzanis 1998). The effect size in that meta-analysis was 0.88 on a measure of executive functioning such as the Wisconsin Card Sorting Test (WCST), and effect sizes ranged from 0.88 for verbal IQ to 1.26 for performance IQ; 0.80 to 1.16 on measures of attention such as Trail Making-B, the Stroop Test, and the Continuous Performance Test (CPT); and 0.41 to 1.41 on measures of secondary verbal memory. In another meta-analysis (Aleman et al. 1999), effect sizes for verbal and nonverbal secondary memory ranged from 0.60 to 1.27, with larger effect sizes for free recall than for recognition memory or cued recall.

Longitudinal Course of Cognitive Performance

The issue of whether there is a course of cognitive decline in pregeriatric adult patients with schizophrenia has been addressed in several older longitudinal studies that have covered approximately 1–14 years between test periods (Haywood and Modelis 1963; Klonoff et al. 1970; Martin et al. 1977; Moran et al. 1962) as reviewed by Randolph et al. (1993). These studies indicated an absence of cognitive deterioration in what has been described as static encephalopathy, but another older study (Schwartzman et al. 1962) showed a deterioration in IQ scores in schizophrenic patients who were more chronically ill but not in those who were not as chronically ill. There also does not appear to be any cognitive deterioration over the first few years of the illness in patients with first-episode schizophrenia (Hoff et al. 1999).

This disassociation in cognitive deterioration between more chronically ill and less chronically ill schizophrenic adult patients is mirrored in elderly schizophrenic patients. Two studies have suggested a further cognitive decline by the seventh decade of life (Davidson et al. 1995, 1996), but this is not an invariant finding because at least one other study (Heaton et al. 1994) showed no difference in cognitive performance between patients with early-onset young, early-onset old, and late-onset schizophrenia. One explanation for the differences in these findings is that the patients in the Heaton et al. (1994) study were less chronically ill than those in the Davidson et al. (1995, 1996) studies. In fact, in one of the studies by Davidson et al. (1995) there was a significant difference in mean (±SD) Mini-Mental State Examination (MMSE) scores from 22.2 (±5.6) in the age range of 25–34 years compared with 9.6 (±7.3) at age 85 years and older in chronically ill patients. Although the older age groups were characterized by a greater degree of negative symptoms, the relationship between negative symptoms and lower MMSE scores was invariant throughout the age ranges. One interesting finding from the study by Harvey et al. (1999) is that geriatric patients with poor outcomes at baseline before cognitive decline are similar to younger schizophrenic patients in that negative symptoms (Addington and Addington 1991; Andreasen and Olsen 1982; McKenna et al. 1989) but not positive symptoms (Addington and Addington 1991; Tamlyn et al. 1992) are related to cognitive impairment. However, over a 30-month period of cognitive decline, whereas negative symptoms were not a risk factor for subsequent cognitive decline, positive symptoms were.

These findings showing a greater cognitive decline in poorer-outcome and more-chronically-ill middle-aged and elderly schizophrenic patients are paralleled by computed tomography findings in younger patients showing progressive increases in ventricular volume in worst-outcome and middle-aged schizophrenic patients (Davis et al. 1998) but not in schizophreniform patients (Jaskiw et al. 1994).

The pattern of cognitive impairment in elderly patients with schizophrenia differs from that of patients with dementia of the Alzheimer's type (DAT). In contrast to DAT, rapid forgetting is absent in schizophrenia (Davidson et al. 1996; Heaton et al. 1994), and there is an encoding and retrieval—as opposed to consolidation—deficit as well as less severe naming and praxis problems (Davidson et al. 1996). Interestingly, on autopsy, elderly schizophrenic patients with dementia do not show a sufficient degree of senile plaques and neurofibrillary tangles to confirm a diagnosis of Alzheimer's disease (AD) or other neurodegenerative disorders (Purohit et al. 1993). Among the candidate neurobiological changes observed in patients with schizophrenia that could account for the cognitive deterioration among the more chronically ill are abnormalities along midline structures or circuits such as the lenticular nuclei (Jernigan et al. 1991), cingulate gyrus, limbic lobe, prefrontal cortices (Weinberger et al. 1992), and medial thalamus (Andreasen et al. 1994). In another sample of elderly institutionalized schizophrenic patients, those with a degree of cognitive impairment that warranted an additional diagnosis of dementia showed reductions in neurotransmitter levels compared with elderly schizophrenic patients without dementia (reduced norepinephrine in the frontal and temporal cortex; Friedman et al. 1999). Such reductions in norepinephrine have been associated with cognitive impairment in patients with AD (Friedman et al. 1999).

Specificity of Cognitive Impairments

Although disturbance in cognitive function is an established feature of chronic schizophrenia (Goldberg et al. 1993a; Kenny and Meltzer 1991; Randolph et al. 1993; Saykin et al. 1991), it does not appear to be specific to schizophrenia; a similar pattern also appears in other psychiatric disorders. For example, several studies have failed to demonstrate a difference in neuropsychological test performance between adult patients with schizophrenia and those with other psychiatric disorders (i.e., bipolar disorder [Hoff et al. 1990; Morice 1990]; bipolar disorder, remitted [Addington and Addington 1997]; affective disorder [bipolar, mixed, and schizoaffective disorder; Rund and Landro 1995]), those with a range of mood disorders including combined unipolar and nonpsychotic bipolar disease (Axelrod et al. 1997), and those with and without psychotic presentations (Silverstein et al. 1994). At least one study (Goldberg et al. 1993a) showed significantly worse performance in schizophrenic patients compared with unipolar and bipolar affective patients. A study of four meta-analyses by Elkis et al. (1995) suggested that this lack of specificity in cognitive impairment between schizophrenia and mood disorders is mirrored in structural brain measures (i.e., ventricular enlargement, increased sulcal prominence).

A few studies suggest that psychosis, independent of diagnosis, may also be an important predictor of neuropsychological test performance. For example, when bipolar patients with and without psychosis are compared with those who have schizophrenia, the bipolar patients with psychosis are no different from schizophrenic patients in terms of test performance. However, bipolar patients without psychosis are less impaired than bipolar patients with psychosis or patients with schizophrenia (Albus et al. 1996; Strauss et al. 1987). Taken together, these findings comparing schizophrenic patients with bipolar patients suggest that symptom presentation (i.e., psychosis) may be a more important predictor of neuropsychological impairment than psychiatric diagnosis.

The fact that positive symptoms are, by and large, unrelated to cognitive performance (Addington and Addington 1991; Tamlyn et al. 1992) is difficult to reconcile with findings suggesting that the presence of psychosis, independently of diagnosis (schizophrenia vs. affective disorders), is more likely to predict neuropsychological impairment than diagnosis per se. This may not be an issue of psychosis being a marker for cognitive impairment under all circumstances but rather of psychosis being more of a marker than diagnosis.

Functional Outcome Implications of Neurocognitive Impairment in Adult Schizophrenia

The functional consequence of neurocognitive deficits in schizophrenia are documented in an extensive review by Green (1996) of 16 available studies described by him as generally "underpowered and exploratory." For example, vigilance was related to social problem solving and skill acquisition, WCST performance to community functioning, and verbal memory to functional outcome, regardless of the measure used. Negative symptoms were also related to social problem solving, but positive symptoms were not significantly associated with outcome measures in any of the studies contained in this review. These findings mirror those described previously in terms of the differing relationship between cognitive measures and negative and positive symptoms.

Green et al. (2000) provided a subsequent update of neurocognitive deficits and functional outcome in adult schizophrenia in which they used a vote-count method as well as a meta-analytic technique to summarize the available studies ($n=37$), which possessed a greater degree of power than those in his previous review. A global cognitive composite score accounted for 48% and 42% of the variance in activities of daily living in two separate patient samples, and when the pathway in the path analysis from cognitive impairment to functional outcome was in the model, direct pathways from psychotic and negative symptoms to functional outcome were not needed (Velligan et al. 1997). This suggests a greater role for neurocognitive impairment than psychopathology in terms of functional outcome. The effect sizes for the composite cognitive measures ranged from small to large (20%–60%). Four separate meta-analyses conducted by Green et al. (2000) on the relationship between functional outcomes measures and more specific cognitive functions indicated that the pooled estimated r weighted by sample size was 0.20 for vigilance, 0.23 for card sorting, 0.29 for secondary verbal memory, and 0.40 for immediate verbal memory, with effect sizes ranging from small to medium for vigilance and from medium to large for immediate verbal memory.

Pharmacological and Cognitive Rehabilitative Treatment of Neurocognitive Impairment in Adult Schizophrenia

In view of the importance of neurocognitive impairment to functional outcome, there has been an increased interest in enhancing neurocognitive integrity pharmacologically and through cognitive rehabilitation techniques, some of which have been borrowed from the head injury literature.

Unfortunately, attempts to pharmacologically improve cognitive functioning in patients with schizophrenia have been thwarted by using medications targeted at psychotic symptoms with myriad side effects rather than by consideration of the underlying neurobiology of the disease and how it affects cognition. This is unlike the use of cholinesterase inhibitors (Evans et al. 2000; Imbibo et al. 2000) in treating cognitive dysfunction in patients with AD, which makes sense given the role of acetylcholine depletion in the basal forebrain and hippocampus and its role in the episodic memory defect in those with AD (Perry et al. 1999).

It is not surprising, therefore, that the cognitive deficits in adult schizophrenia, with a few exceptions, tend to be relatively refractory to both typical (Cassens et al. 1990) and atypical medications such as clozapine (Goldberg et al. 1993c; Hagger et al. 1993). However, recent reviews (Keefe et al. 1999; Meltzer and McGurk 1999; Purdon 2000) and reports (Green et al. 1997; Kern et al. 1999) of other atypical drugs (e.g., olanzapine and risperidone) suggest more promising trends in terms of atypical antipsychotic interventions. The meta-analysis of Keefe et al. (1999) showed that atypical antipsychotic medications, when compared with typical antipsychotic drugs, improved verbal fluency, digit-symbol substitution, fine motor functions, executive functions, and to a lesser degree, attention. Learning and memory functions were the least responsive, but risperidone was found in another study (Kern et al. 1999) to improve verbal learning and secondary memory compared with haloperidol. Risperidone was also found to improve verbal working memory compared with haloperidol (Green et al. 1997). However, as noted by Keefe et al. (1999), "in no study did the cognitive functions of patients with schizophrenia reach normal levels" (p. 211). Also, there appears to have been too great an emphasis placed on statistically significant improvements in cognition after pharmacotherapy and too little emphasis on clinical significance. For example, in the study by Green et al. (1997), there was only a 13% improvement in verbal working memory compared with the pre-drug baseline.

Appropriately, it has been noted by Purdon (2000) that "strong statements about the relative and differential efficacy of the novel medications would be premature" (p. 110) because of issues such as most comparisons' not being double blind and differences in sample size, measurement techniques, and statistical analyses. Moreover, most studies on the effect of atypical antipsychotic agents on cognition have been carried out with more chronic schizophrenic patient samples. However, at least one study (Purdon et al. 2000) used patients with early-phase schizophrenia and showed that olanzapine, relative to haloperidol or risperidone, showed improvement on immediate recall and on the Hooper Visual Organization Test. Of note, these were only two of 17 cognitive measures to improve after a Bonferroni adjustment, suggesting minimal overall improvement in neurocognitive dysfunction. In another study, after 1 year of treatment with a typical neuroleptic drug, patients with first-episode schizophrenia exhibited an improvement in attention, verbal learning, and verbal memory compared with the untreated baseline condition (Bilder et al. 1991). However, on balance, there was a high level of stability over this period in neuropsychological deficits during acute and long-term treatment. Taken together, these findings suggest relatively greater improvement on memory after typical and atypical neuroleptic treatment than has been previously reported for samples of patients with chronic schizophrenia (Cassens et al. 1990).

This relative refractoriness of cognitive dysfunction suggests an enduring and trait-like, rather than state-like, phenomenon. It could also suggest, as mentioned, that the appropriate neurobiological substrate for cognitive dysfunction in patients with schizophrenia has not been targeted by even the atypical antipsychotic medications, which also have side effects and complex interactions among the side effects that can adversely affect cognition (Keefe et al. 1999).

The failure of neuropsychological deficits to improve or normalize in the previously mentioned studies with either typical or atypical antipsychotic medication, despite an improvement in psychotic symptoms, provides further evidence of the dissociation between psychotic symptoms and cognitive dysfunction in schizophrenia, at least in terms of the targets of the pharmacological manipulations. This is consistent with the findings that show that, independent of treatment effects, a significant relationship exists between cognitive impairment and negative symptoms (Addington and Addington 1991; Andreasen and Olsen 1982; McKenna et al. 1989) but not positive (psychotic) symptoms (Addington and Addington 1991; Tamlyn et al. 1992) in schizophrenia.

As for cognitive impairment being refractory to antipsychotic medications, other factors exist above and beyond not having pharmacologically targeted the appropriate neurobiological substrate for cognition. This may may simply reflect a separate issue—that is, that cognitive symptoms in schizophrenia reflect a type of brain dysfunction that is not amenable to antipsychotic drug treatment. Alternatively, negative symptoms such as apathy and anhedonia, which are also less responsive to pharmacotherapy than positive symptoms (Hagger et al. 1993), could still be exercising an adverse impact on cognition after such treatment. As noted, medication side effects, their complex interactions, and the complex interactions among neurotransmitter systems—some of which worsen cognition (Keefe et al. 1999)—could be rate-limiting factors in attempts to enhance cognition.

An alternative, or adjunctive, intervention to psychopharmacological manipulation is that of cognitive rehabilitation. Many of the issues and controversies about cognitive rehabilitation in schizophrenia, such as failure to generalize beyond the training task and minimal clinical significance, have already been addressed in the head injury literature (Gordon 1990; Ruff et al. 1993). Strategies vary from repetitious practicing of impaired functions to developing compensatory techniques to bypass the impaired functions. Memory retraining of brain-damaged patients also has a long history (Wilson and Moffat 1992), with techniques varying from repetitive recall drills to mnemonic strategy training to the use of prosthetic devices (Sohlberg et al. 1992).

An interesting innovation attempted in the rehabilitation of cognitive dysfunction in schizophrenia is "errorless learning." This technique involves the elimination of trial-and-error learning in that the patients begin with very easy discriminations and do not experience failure. Task difficulty is only gradually increased. The rationale for this was delineated in a study by Baddeley and Wilson (1994) of amnesic patients that showed this technique to be more effective than traditional "effortful" trial-and-error learning because in trial-and-error learning errors are implicitly remembered, which interferes with the retrieval of target items (O'Carroll et al. 1999). In the field of memory rehabilitation, the emphasis has been on "effortful" approaches and, according to O'Carroll et al. (1999), this is predicated on the "levels of processing" conceptualization of Craik and Lockhart (1972), wherein "working hard" on the material to be remembered enhances the depth of encoding and efficiency of retention and retrieval. As a result, the emphasis in much of the cognitive rehabilitation literature has been on enhancing declarative or explicit memory as opposed to procedural or implicit memory.

More recent studies have shown enhanced memory (O'Carroll et al. 1999) and WCST performance (Kern et al. 1996) in patients with schizophrenia using this errorless learning paradigm. Everyday procedural activities such as keyboard skills can also be effectively trained using this procedure (Baddeley and Wilson 1994). A combination of procedural and errorless learning, targeted reinforcement, and massed practice appears to facilitate cognitive flexibility and memory in patients with schizophrenia (Wykes et al. 1999).

As pointed out by Bellack et al. (1999), although certain cognitive measures are related to functional outcome measures,

> [t]he accumulated findings provide clear evidence that performance can be enhanced on a range of cognitive tasks through practice, instruction, and provision of incentives...the gains achieved in these studies do not appear to have had large clinical effects on other aspects of functioning...or to higher level domains (e.g., social skills). (p. 262)

Again, this raises the issue of the limited generalizability of cognitive remediation techniques that was mentioned previously and was demonstrated by the failure of schizophrenic patients to show generalizability from enhanced performance on the WCST to the Category Test after training (Bellack et al. 1999).

There are multiple possible causes for this failure to generalize, including the fact that "social performance in the community depends upon a number of factors in addition to having the capacity to perform a behavior in controlled circumstances, such as motivation to engage in social interaction and prior experience in similar encounters" (Bellack et al. 1999, p. 259). Also, cognitive rehabilitation strategies need to be individualized to a much greater extent, especially given the variability in performance across both individuals and different cognitive functions in schizophrenia (Bellack et al. 1999), and there needs to be much greater emphasis on the development of compensatory strategies using individuals' cognitive strengths as opposed to practice-based, repetitive types of training targeted at improving their areas of cognitive weakness (Bellack et al. 1999).

Early-Stage Schizophrenia

The presence of cognitive impairment in young and middle-aged patients with chronic schizophrenia, along with an absence of cognitive decline over the course of middle-adult years after the onset of the illness and after chronicity takes hold (Goldberg et al. 1993b; Haywood and Modelis 1963; Klonoff et al. 1970; Martin et al. 1977; Moran et al. 1962), has led to a renewed focus on earlier stages of cognitive impairment in schizophrenia. As noted in the introductory section, *stage* can mean either stage of chronological development or stage of illness onset. Several important and interrelated issues exist regarding early-stage schizophrenia. The first is whether the cognitive abnormalities are present premorbidly (i.e., before the onset of psychosis) and, if so, when during development they emerge. The second is whether psychosis onset causes or worsens the cognitive abnormalities (or both). The third issue is whether early-onset schizophrenia is a more virulent form of the disease than later-onset forms and therefore results in more profound cognitive impairment.

First-Episode Adult Schizophrenia

Cognitive impairment appears to be present at least as early as the first episode in adult patients with schizophrenia (Bilder et al. 1991; Hoff et al. 1991; Saykin et al. 1994). Several studies have shown that within the first year and soon after the first break, patients with schizophrenia manifest impaired performance in verbal learning, verbal recall, and verbal fluency. Despite some improvement in cognition after 1 year of treatment with a typical neuroleptic drug, on balance there was a high level of stability over this period of time in neuropsychological deficits during acute and long-term treatment (Bilder et al. 1991). As mentioned previously, these findings appear to show relatively greater improvement on memory after typical neuroleptic treatment than has been previously reported for samples of patients with more chronic schizophrenia (Cassens et al. 1990).

The data regarding stability in neuropsychological test performance within the first 1–2 years of illness in adult patients with schizophrenia have provided somewhat discrepant findings. Some cross-sectional studies comparing patients with early-stage schizophrenia with those with chronic schizophrenia suggest a deterioration (Bilder et al. 1995; Schwartzman and Douglas 1962). Although Saykin et al. (1994) showed that, compared with chronic schizophrenic patients from an earlier study (Saykin et al. 1991), first-episode patients were significantly less impaired on measures of attention and visual memory and marginally less impaired on measures of verbal learning and memory, the overall shape of the cognitive profiles reflective of degrees of impairment by cognitive domain revealed no difference between these patient groups. Another cross-sectional study (Hoff et al. 1991) suggested stability of neuropsychological impairment. Because these studies employed cross-sectional designs, reported cognitive differences may have been caused by sample bias effects as opposed to developmental trends. In terms of longitudinal designs with first-episode schizophrenic patients, one study indicated a rapid decline in cognition within the first 6 months (Bilder et al. 1991); another indicated improvements over a 1- or 2-year follow-up period (Hoff et al. 1992); and yet another indicated stability (Hoff et al. 1999). As mentioned previously, studies that use longitudinal designs over approximately 1–14 years have indicated an absence of deterioration or static encephalopathy (Haywood and Modelis 1963; Klonoff et al. 1970; Martin et al. 1977; Moran et al. 1962), at least with respect to less chronic adult pregeriatric schizophrenia.

Adolescent-Onset Versus Adult-Onset Schizophrenia

It has been postulated that adolescent-onset schizophrenia is a distinctive, and perhaps more virulent, subtype of the disease (Gillberg et al. 1993; Johnstone et al. 1989; Kolakowska et al. 1985; McClellan et al. 1993). Consistent with this formulation, Johnstone et al. (1989) used a limited selection of cognitive tests and found that patients with adolescent-onset schizophrenia had poorer remote memory (i.e., recall of events from the distant past) than those with adult-onset schizophrenia. In using a more comprehensive neuropsychological test battery, Basso et al. (1997) were able to confirm these findings by showing that, in contrast to patients with adult-onset schizophrenia, adults patients with adolescent-onset schizophrenia exhibited more severely impaired performance on a broad range of cognitive measures, especially memory and executive functions.

Although the adolescent-onset group had longer durations of illness, this variable was significantly related to only two of the neuropsychological measures. None of the measures on which the adolescent-onset patients performed more poorly than the adult-onset group were significantly related to illness duration.

Adolescents With Schizophrenia

The onset of schizophrenia frequently occurs during adolescence (Beratis et al. 1994; Häfner et al. 1982; Loranger 1984). Despite this, there are relatively few studies of this population (for review, see Findling et al. 1995). This is in marked contrast to the vast literature on adult schizophrenia, both in terms of first-episode (Bilder et al. 1991; Hoff et al. 1991; Saykin et al. 1994) and chronic schizophrenia (Kenny and Meltzer 1991; Randolph et al. 1993; Saykin et al. 1991).

The adolescent years are of particular interest because of convergent evidence for important neurodevelopmental changes during this period. Primate and human studies indicate changes in synaptic density and morphology in the frontal lobe (Feinberg et al. 1990; Huttenlocher 1979; Lewis et al. 1995). Human studies have indicated that during this same period of development, there is a decline in the ratio of gray matter to white matter (Jernigan and Tallal 1990) as well as a marked decline in the duration of stage 4 sleep (slow wave, non–rapid eye movement) and amplitude of delta electroencephalographic waves (Feinberg et al. 1990). Positron emission tomography studies indicate a decline in glucose metabolism from childhood to adolescence (Chugani et al. 1987). These changes have been conceptualized as involving maturational reorganization consisting of selective synaptic enhancement and elimination of redundant axons (i.e., pruning). These maturational events have been summoned in support of what Keshaven et al. (1994) have described as a "late" neurodevelopmental model of the etiology of schizophrenia (Feinberg 1983; Feinberg et al. 1990) in contrast to the "early" developmental model, which posits a fixed lesion from early life that interacts with normal neurodevelopmental events occurring at a later point (Murray et al. 1988; Weinberger 1987).

The neuropsychological functioning of adolescent patients with schizophrenia remains largely unexamined, and studies that have been conducted have generally not compared patients with normal control subjects or have not used a battery assessing a range of cognitive functions. Thus, Erickson et al. (1984) found no evidence for attentional impairments in schizophrenic patients compared with other psychiatric patients (mostly those with attention-deficit disorder) on the Continuous Performance Test. Gottschalk and Selin (1991) found that compared with other adolescent psychiatric patients (mostly depressed), adolescent schizophrenic patients with conduct disorder (referred to by the authors as the "probable schizophrenia group") exhibited impaired performance on the Rhythm Test (interpreted as an attentional task by the authors) and the Halstead Category Test, a measure of abstract reasoning and executive functions. Finally, Goldberg et al. (1988) showed a lowered performance IQ, but not a lowered verbal IQ, in psychotic adolescent patients compared with nonpsychotic adolescent psychiatric control subjects.

Because there is a paucity of studies directly related to adolescent patients with schizophrenia, it was deemed important by our research group to extend the findings of previous investigators (Erickson et al. 1984; Goldberg et al. 1988; Gottschalk and Selin 1991) by comparing the neuropsychological test performance of adolescent patients with schizophrenia with that of age-matched control subjects on a range of measures of cognitive functioning found to be impaired in patients with adult first-episode (Bilder et al. 1991; Hoff et al. 1991; Saykin et al. 1994) as well as chronic (Saykin et al. 1991; Kenny and Meltzer 1991; Randolph et al. 1993) schizophrenia.

Overall, the adolescent patients with schizophrenia in our study (Kenny et al. 1997) exhibited a pattern of neuropsychological deficits similar to that of patients with first-episode (Bilder et al. 1991; Hoff et al. 1991; Saykin et al. 1994) and chronic (Kenny and Meltzer 1991; Randolph et al. 1993; Saykin et al. 1991) schizophrenia. Accordingly, they manifested deficits in divided attention (Digit Span Distraction and Stroop Test), short-term or working memory (recalling consonant trigrams after 15 seconds of counting backwards), recent long-term memory (list learning recall, prose recall, and recognition memory for words), and executive functions (WCST percent perseverative errors). There was also a trend toward impaired performance on the Paced Auditory Serial Addition Test, the Digit Symbol Test of the Wechsler Intelligence Scale for Children–Revised (WISC-R), and the Category Instance Generation Test. By contrast, there was no evidence of impaired performance on the Controlled Oral Word Association Test, the WISC-R Maze Test, or the Judgment of Line Orientation Test.

The fact that there was no difference in performance on WISC-R estimates of IQ suggests that the cognitive deficits in adolescent patients with schizophrenia are not caused by a global cognitive dysfunction. These findings also suggest that crystallized (WISC-R verbal IQ) and fluid (performance IQ) aspects of intelligence are relatively intact. However, this finding is at variance with the findings of Goldberg et al. (1988), who showed a lowered performance IQ but not a lowered verbal IQ in psychotic adolescent patients compared with nonpsychotic adolescent psychiatric control subjects. Performance in our sample of adolescent schizophrenic patients was also unimpaired on the Judgment of Line Orientation Test, Controlled Oral Word Association Test, and Category Instance Generation Test, providing further support for unimpaired visuospatial and language functions. It is also noteworthy that because the patients were sufficiently stabilized on antipsychotic medication to function on an outpatient basis, their cognitive deficits were not likely secondary to significant psychotic disruption. The cognitive deficits may be an expression of compromised brain integrity as evidenced by the findings of Schulz et al. (1983), which showed enlarged ventricles and sulcal prominence in adolescents with schizophrenia. A relationship has been demonstrated between neuropsychological test performance and structural measures of brain abnormality in adult patients with chronic (Donnelly et al. 1980; Golden et al. 1980) and first-episode (Bilder et al. 1995) schizophrenia.

These findings are important in demonstrating that the cognitive deficits associated with schizophrenia occur at an earlier developmental stage rather than after a prolonged course of decline such as occurs in DAT (Lezak 1983). Whether these deficits are of the magnitude shown by adult patients with schizophrenia is not known. A comparison of effect sizes with those from a previously published study (Hagger et al. 1993) showed that effect sizes were larger for some cognitive measures in the chronic sample. However, any attempt to compare adolescent patients with adult patients in a cross-sectional design is fraught with peril because of the aforementioned limitations of a cross-sectional design, such as sample bias and the psychosocial and other consequences of chronic illness. What makes this even more problematic in adolescents is the fact that the normal control subjects are also undergoing developmental changes in cognition during this period. In fact, comparison of the control adolescent subjects with control subjects from a previous study (Hagger et al. 1993) indicated such a trend with respect to performance on language (Category Instance Generation) and reasoning (WCST) tasks. What can be said, however, is that the pattern of impaired and unimpaired neuropsychological test performance is consistent with that previously reported for adult patients with chronic, treatment-resistant schizophrenia (Hagger et al. 1993).

Children With Schizophrenia

A recent review by Jacobsen and Rapoport (1998) noted that neuropsychological deficits are evident in children with schizophrenia. These are particularly prominent on tasks that involve fine motor speed and demand attention or require short-term memory capacity (Asarnow et al. 1994, 1995).

By contrast, basic visuospatial functioning, such as judging the angular orientation of radiating lines and as assessed by the Judgment of Line Orientation Test, has been shown to be unimpaired (Schneider and Asarnow 1987). The verbal comprehension factor, which includes the Information, Similarities, Vocabulary, and Comprehension subtests of the WISC-R, was also unimpaired, as was the perceptual organizational factor (Asarnow et al. 1987).

This pattern of impaired and unimpaired neuropsychological functions is consistent with that reported for patients with chronic and first-episode schizophrenia as well as for adolescents with schizophrenia. Again, given the absence of longitudinal test data, it is difficult to determine the extent to which these patient populations differ in terms of magnitude of cognitive impairment.

In summary, the preponderance of evidence suggests that cognitive impairment in patients with schizophrenia is evident early in the course of the illness, with little progressive decline over the middle adult years, except in more-chronic patient samples in the middle adult years and in some elderly patients.

Prepsychotic Cognitive Functioning in Schizophrenia

Children who may be at risk for developing schizophrenia (i.e., those with parents who have schizophrenia) show deficits in information processing (see Nuechterlein and Dawson 1984 for review). The problem with methodology is that data are not yet available as to how many of these children have actually gone on to develop schizophrenia.

More promising are retrospective studies of cognitive and academic performance of children who subsequently develop schizophrenia. These have generally indicated lowered intellect compared with children who did not develop schizophrenia (Aylward et al. 1984). These studies were not population based, however, and many used outdated concepts of schizophrenia.

The most definitive examinations of this issue are population-based longitudinal studies in which data are available on individuals who have actually gone on to develop schizophrenia, such as are represented in the British population cohort studies (e.g., the Medical Research Council National Survey of Health and Development [NSHD] and National Child Development Study [NCDS]). These have been extensively reviewed by Jones (1997). These were longitudinal studies conducted to address the issue of whether childhood IQ or school performance (or both) before the onset of psychosis predicts the subsequent development of schizophrenia.

Of the 4,746 individuals in the NSHD study alive in the United Kingdom at age 16 years, 30 met DSM-III-R criteria for schizophrenia or schizoaffective disorder. In the NCDS study, composed of 15,398 persons age 7 years, 15,303 age 9 years, 14,761 age 16 years, and 12,537 age 23 years, 29 individuals received a Present State Examination (PSE)/ CATEGO diagnosis of narrow schizophrenia. In the NSHD study, children who later developed schizophrenia attained lower IQ scores at ages 11 and 15 years. Similar results were shown in the NCDS study, in which, at ages 7 and 11 years, children who later developed schizophrenia performed more poorly than control subjects on a wide range of tasks, including general IQ, oral ability, and quality of speech. Crystallized aspects of intelligence were as deficient as fluid intelligence, suggesting a diffuse and global type impairment. As with adults, these deficits may not be unique as these developmental differences have also been shown, albeit to a lesser degree, in those who develop chronic affective illness (i.e., depression) (van Os et al. 1997).

Analysis of the NHSD and NCDS data by Jones and Done (1997) revealed no evidence of bimodality in the distribution of IQ scores between patients and control subjects or within the case group itself. Scores for the majority of cases were within 2 standard deviations of the control mean values. According to Jones (1997), these findings argue against a particularly deviant developmental subtype of schizophrenia and in favor of "the majority of children destined to develop schizophrenia showing a slight decrement in IQ, thereby shifting the entire distribution and resulting in a lower group mean" (p. 143).

In another study, the 10% of individuals with larger-than-expected IQ declines from ages 4–7 had a rate of psychosis by the age of 23 years that was almost seven times that of those that did not exhibit such a prepsychotic cognitive decline (Kremen et al. 1998). Consistent with these findings are those of David et al. (1997), which showed a highly significant association between low IQ scores at age 18 years and the subsequent development of schizophrenia. This study also demonstrated that, in addition to global impairment (IQ) as a predictor of the development of schizophrenia, there was an additional risk conferred by specific cognitive deficits (i.e., mechanical knowledge and, to a lesser extent, verbal IQ).

These results are consistent with those reported by Jones et al. (1994), who found an association between low educational test scores at ages 8, 11, and 15 and the later development of schizophrenia. As mentioned, low IQ scores at ages 11 and 15 years were also associated with the later development of schizophrenia.

Pre- Versus Postpsychotic Cognitive Functioning in Schizophrenia

Evidence very clearly shows that cognitive deficits precede the onset of psychosis in schizophrenia. The question still remains as to whether the cognitive deficits in schizophrenia are exacerbated by early-stage psychotic events. Comparisons of pre- and postmorbid cognitive performance in adult patients with schizophrenia have indicated deteriorations in performance (Lubin et al. 1962; Schwartzman and Douglas 1962) within several years of illness onset. However, one study (Albee et al. 1963) was not able to replicate these findings, and another (Hamlin 1969) showed an increase in IQ over time. A more recent study (Russell et al. 1997) compared the prepsychotic IQs of children (mean age, 13.3±3.1 years) with their postpsychotic IQ scores as adults with schizophrenia (mean age, 32.9±3.2 years) and found no evidence of a deterioration in IQ scores.

Taken together, the findings of deterioration effects after psychosis onset are clearly less compelling than the findings of prepsychotic cognitive dysfunction in schizophrenia. The evidence is also more compellingly in favor of a neurodevelopmental hypothesis, with possibly some later-onset decline in a subset of more chronically ill patients.

Etiology of Early-Stage
Cognitive Dysfunction in Schizophrenia

Although the early-stage prepsychotic cognitive dysfunction in patients with schizophrenia argues in favor of a neurodevelopmental hypothesis, it is not entirely clear whether this represents a neurobiological phenomenon or is a reflection of prodromal factors such as social withdrawal. Thus, social behavioral difficulties may have lowered IQ scores independently of neurodevelopmental brain processes. As such, low IQ scores may merely be another prodromal expression. Arguing against such an interpretation is the finding of David et al. (1997), which showed that adjusting for such factors did not have an appreciable attenuating effect on the relationship between low IQ and the development of schizophrenia. The fact that the relationship between low IQ and the subsequent development of schizophrenia is evident before the prodromal stage also argues against low IQ being caused by prodromal factors (Jones 1997; Kremen et al. 1998).

Early fetal abnormalities of either a genetic or neurobiological environmental (obstetric complications) origin have also been implicated in the development of schizophrenia (Jones and Murray 1991). The fact that the relationship between IQ and the development of schizophrenia remained after adjustment for genetic effects (i.e., family history of schizophrenia) argues against an exclusively genetic etiology (David et al. 1997). Similarly, when genetic risk is controlled, such as in the Goldberg et al. (1990) study on monozygotic twins discordant for schizophrenia, the association between schizophrenia and IQ remained. David et al. (1997), citing the Geddes and Lawrie (1995) study, commented that "obstetric complications confer an approximately two-fold risk of schizophrenia only and so are unlikely to entirely account for the strength of association [between low IQ and the development of schizophrenia] here" (p. 1321).

Because the positive predictive power of low IQ is insufficient to entirely predict the subsequent development of schizophrenia, low IQ by itself is not likely to increase such risk (David et al. 1997). The fact that the risk factors (e.g., obstetric and birth complications) for the development of schizophrenia are correlated with IQ suggested to David et al. (1997) that "lowered IQ could be the means by which other genetic or environmental [obstetric complications] influences increase the risk of schizophrenia" (p. 1321).

Recent neuropathological evidence suggests a role for neurobiological factors as underlying the neurodevelopmental cognitive abnormalities observed in those with early-stage schizophrenia. For example, there has been a conspicuous lack of gliosis in the brains of patients with schizophrenia (Jones 1997). Gliosis is the neural scarring that results from lesions other than those that take place during early development. Second, neuroimaging abnormalities, particularly ventricular enlargement, have been demonstrated at the outset of psychosis (Turner et al. 1986) during adolescence (Schulz et al. 1983) and appear not to be progressive (Jaskiw et al. 1994) except in worst-outcome middle-aged schizophrenic patients (Davis et al. 1998).

As with IQ, attempts to identify bimodality in the distributions of enlarged ventricles have failed (Daniels et al. 1991; Harvey et al. 1990). Rather, the whole population of patients with schizophrenia appears to be shifted relative to control subjects. There was a very evident linear relationship between ventricular volume and risk of schizophrenia, as was the case with IQ in the two British cohort studies.

Conclusions

The presence of cognitive impairment across the developmental spectrum in schizophrenia (i.e., children before and after psychosis onset, adolescence, first-episode young adult, and adult chronic patients) argues in favor of a neurodevelopmental explanation of such deficits. The absence of cognitive decline in less chronic samples over the course of middle adult years after the onset of the illness and after chronicity takes hold argues against a neurodegenerative hypothesis in theses samples, but there does appear to be some cognitive deterioration, especially in elderly, more chronic patients. As noted previously, "early stage" can mean either stage of chronological development or stage of illness onset.

There are a number of important and interrelated issues regarding early-stage schizophrenia. The first issue is whether the cognitive abnormalities are present premorbidly (before the onset of psychosis). The data reviewed in this chapter very clearly indicate that cognitive deficits (e.g., low IQ) before the onset of psychosis are predictive of the development of schizophrenia. These deficits appear to be present from very early ages (4–7 years) and continue throughout prepubescent (age 11) and adolescent (ages 15–18) stages of chronological development.

The evidence of a worsening of cognitive functioning after the onset of psychosis is less compelling than is the evidence for the existence of cognitive deficits before the onset of psychosis.

Early-onset schizophrenia appears to be a more virulent form of the disease than later-onset schizophrenia and, therefore, results in more profound cognitive impairment.

The fact that the risk factors for the development of schizophrenia (e.g., obstetric and birth complications) are correlated with IQ suggested to David et al. (1997) that "lowered IQ could be the means by which other genetic or environmental influences increase the risk of schizophrenia" (p. 1321).

Recent neuropathological evidence suggests that a neurobiological etiological factor underlies the neurodevelopmental cognitive abnormalities observed in patients with early-stage schizophrenia. These include a conspicuous lack of gliosis in the brains of schizophrenic patients (which argues against a later developmental lesion) and neuroimaging abnormalities, particularly ventricular enlargement, that have been demonstrated at the outset of psychosis as well as during adolescence and appear not to be progressive except in more chronic patients.

The fact that cognitive abnormalities are present during childhood and adolescence indicates that academic or learning difficulties are likely to present themselves long before the onset of psychosis. The findings from the study by Kenny et al. (1997) demonstrating cognitive impairment in remitted adolescent patients with schizophrenia indicate that treatment with antipsychotic medication is likely to have little beneficial impact on cognitive functioning in such patients. This is consistent with what has been found in patients with chronic adult schizophrenia.

References

Addington J, Addington D: Positive and negative symptoms of schizophrenia: their course and relationship over time. Schizophr Res 5:51–59, 1991

Addington J, Addington D: Attentional vulnerability in schizophrenia and bipolar disorder. Schizophr Res 23:197–204, 1997

Albee G, Corcoran C, Werneke A: Childhood and intercurrent intellectual performance of adult schizophrenics. J Consult Clin Psychol 27:364–366, 1963

Albus M, Hubman W, Wahlheim C, et al: Acta Psychiatr Scand 94:87–93, 1996

Aleman A, Hijman R, de Hann EHF, et al: Memory impairment in schizophrenia: a meta-analysis. Am J Psychiatry 156:1358–1366, 1999

Andreasen NC, Olsen S: Negative vs positive schizophrenia: definition and validation. Arch Gen Psychiatry 39:789–794, 1982

Andreasen NC, Arndt S, Swayze V II, et al: Thalamic abnormalities in schizophrenia visualized through magnetic resonance imaging averaging. Science 266:294–298, 1994

Asarnow RF, Tanguay PE, Bott L, et al: Patterns of intellectual functioning in non-retarded autistic and schizophrenic children. J Child Psychol Psychiatry 28:273–280, 1987

Asarnow RF, Asamen J, Granholm E, et al: Cognitive/neuropsychological studies of children with a schizophrenic disorder. Schizophr Bull 20:647–669, 1994

Asarnow RF, Brown W, Strandburg R: Children with a schizophrenic disorder: neurobehavioral studies. Eur Arch Psychiatry Clin Neurosci 245:70–79, 1995

Axelrod BN, Goldman RS, Tompkins LM, et al: Differential patterns performance on the Wisconsin Card Sorting Test in schizophrenia, mood disorder, and traumatic brain injury. Neuropsychiatry Neuropsychol Behav Neurol 7:20–24, 1997

Aylward E, Walker E, Bettes B: Intelligence in schizophrenia: meta-analysis of the research. Schizophr Bull 10:430–459, 1984

Baddeley A, Wilson BA: When implicit memory learning fails: amnesia and the problem of error elimination. Neuropsychologia 32:53–68, 1994

Basso MR, Nasrallah HA, Olson SC, et al: Cognitive deficits distinguish patients with adolescent-onset and adult-onset schizophrenia. Neuropsychol Behav Neurol 10:107–112, 1997

Bellack AS, Gold JM, Buchanin RW: Cognitive rehabilitation for schizophrenia: problems, prospects, and strategies. Schizophr Bull 25:257–274, 1999

Beratis S, Gabriel J, Hoidas S: Age at onset in subtypes of schizophrenic disorders. Schizophr Bull 20:287–296, 1994

Bilder RM, Kipschultz-Broch L, Reiter G, et al: Neuropsychological studies of first episode schizophrenia. Schizophr Res 4:381–382, 1991

Bilder RM, Bogerts B, Ashtari M, et al: Anterior hippocampal volume reductions predict frontal lobe dysfunction in first episode schizophrenia. Schizophr Res 17:47–58, 1995

Cassens G, Inglis AK, Appelbaum PS, et al: Neuroleptics: effects on neuropsychological functions in chronic schizophrenic patients. Schizophr Bull 16:477–499, 1990

Chugani HT, Phelps ME, Mazziotta JC: Positron emission tomography study of human brain functional development. Ann Neurol 22:487–497, 1987

Craik FIM, Lockhart RS: Levels of processing: a framework for memory research. J Verb Learn Verb Behav 11:671–684, 1972

Daniels DG, Goldberg TE, Gibbons RD, et al: Lack of bimodal distribution of ventricular size in schizophrenia: a Gaussian mixture analysis of 1056 cases and controls. Biol Psychiatry 30:887–903, 1991

David AS, Malmberg A, Brandt L, et al: IQ and risk for schizophrenia: a population-based cohort study. Psychol Med 27:1311–1323, 1997

Davidson M, Harvey P, Welsh KA, et al: Severity of symptoms in chronically institutionalized geriatric schizophrenic patients. Am J Psychiatry 152:197–207, 1995

Davidson M, Harvey P, Welsh KA, et al: Cognitive functioning in late-life schizo-phrenia: a comparison of elderly schizophrenic patients and patients with Alzheimer's disease. Am J Psychiatry 153:1274–1279, 1996

Davis KL, Buchsbaum MS, Shihabuddin L: Ventricular enlargement in poor outcome schizophrenia. Biol Psychiatry 43:783–793, 1998

Donnelly EF, Weinberger DR, Waldman IN, et al: Cognitive impairment associated with morphological brain abnormalities on computerized tomography in chronic schizophrenic patients. J Nerv Ment Dis 168:305–308, 1980

Elkis H, Friedman L, Wise A, et al: Meta-analyses of studies of ventricular enlarge-ment and cortical sulcal prominence in mood disorders: comparison with controls or patients with schizophrenia. Arch Gen Psychiatry 52:735–746, 1995

Erickson WD, Yellin AM, Hopwood JH, et al: The effects of neuroleptics in attention in adolescent schizophrenics. Biol Psychiatry 19:745–753, 1984

Evans M, Ellis A, Watson D, et al: Sustained cognitive improvement following treatment of Alzheimer's disease with donepezil. Int J Geriatr Psychiatry 15:50–53, 2000

Feinberg I: Schizophrenia: caused by a fault in programmed synaptic elimination during adolescence? J Psychiatry Res 17:319–334, 1983

Feinberg I, Thode HC, Chugani HT, et al: Gamma distribution model describes maturational curves for delta wave amplitude, cortical metabolic rate and synaptic density. J Theor Biol 142:149–161, 1990

Findling RL, Friedman L, Kenny JT, et al: Adolescent schizophrenia: a methodologic review of the current neuroimaging and neuropsychologic literature. J Autism Develop Dis 25:627–639, 1995

Friedman JI, Temporini H, Davis KL: Pharmacologic strategies for augmenting cognitive performance in schizophrenia. Biol Psychiatry 45:1–16, 1999

Geddes JR, Lawrie SM: Obstetric complications and schizophrenia: a meta-analysis. Br J Psychiatry 167:786–793, 1995

Gillberg IC, Hellgren L, Gillberg C: Psychotic disorders diagnosed in adolescence: outcome at age 30 years. J Child Psychol Psychiatry 34:1173–1185, 1993

Goldberg TE, Karson CN, Leleszi JP, et al: Intellectual impairment in adolescent psychosis: a controlled parametric study. Schizophr Res 1:261–266, 1988

Goldberg TE, Raglund DR, Gold J, et al: Neuropsychological assessment of monozy-gotic twins discordant for schizophrenia. Arch Gen Psychiatry 47:1066–1072, 1990

Goldberg TE, Gold JM, Greenberg R, et al: Contrast between patients with affective disorders and schizophrenia on a neuropsychological test battery. Am J Psy-chiatry 150:1355–1362, 1993a

Goldberg TE, Hyde TM, Kleinman JE, et al: Course of schizophrenia: neuropsy-chological evidence for at static encephalophathy. Schizophr Bull 19:797–804, 1993b

Goldberg TE, Greenberg RD, Griffin SJ, et al: The impact of clozapine on cognition and psychiatric symptoms in patients with schizophrenia. Br J Psychiatry 162:43–48, 1993c

Golden CJ, Moses JA, Zelazowski R, et al: Cerebral ventricular size and neuropsychological impairment in young chronic schizophrenics. Arch Gen Psychiatry 37:619–623, 1980

Gordon WA: Cognitive remediation: an approach to the amelioration of behavioral disorders, in Neurobehavioral Sequelae of Traumatic Brain Injury. Edited by Wood RLI. New York, Taylor & Francis, 1990, pp 175–193

Gottschalk LA, Selin C: Comparative neurobiological and neuropsychological deficits in adolescent and adult schizophrenic and nonschizophrenic patients. Psychother Psychosom 55:32–41, 1991

Green MF: What are the functional consequences of neurocognitive deficits in schizophrenia? Am J Psychiatry 153:321–330, 1996

Green MF, Marshall Jr BD, Wirshing WC, et al: Does risperidone improve verbal working memory in treatment-resistant schizophrenia? Am J Psychiatry 154:799–804, 1997

Green MF, Kern RS, Braff DJ, et al: Neurocognitive deficits and functional outcomes: are we measuring the "right stuff?" Schizophr Bull 26:119–136, 2000

Hafner H, Riechler-Rossler A, Maurer K, et al: First onset and early symptomatology of schizophrenia: a chapter of epidemiological and neurobiological research into age and sex differences. Eur Arch Psychiatry Clin Neurosci 242:109–118, 1992

Hagger C, Buckley P, Kenny JT, et al: Improvement in cognitive functions and psychiatric symptoms in treatment-resistant schizophrenic patients receiving clozapine. Biol Psychiatry 34:702–712, 1993

Hamlin R: The stability of intellectual function in chronic schizophrenia. J Nerv Ment Dis 149:495–503, 1969

Harvey I, McGuffen P, Williams M, et al: The ventricle-brain ration (VBR) in functional psychosis: an admixture analysis. Psychiatry Res 35:61–69, 1990

Harvey PD, Earle-Boyer EA, Wieglus MS, et al: Encoding, memory, and thought disorder in schizophrenia and mania. Schizophr Bull 12:252–261, 1999

Haywood HC, Modelis I: Effect of symptom change on intellectual function in schizophrenia. J Abnorm Soc Psychol 67:76–78, 1963

Heaton R, Paulsen JS, McAdams LA, et al: Neuropsychological deficits in schizophrenia: relationship to age, chronicity, and dementia. Arch Gen Psychiatry 51:469–476, 1994

Heinrichs RW, Zakzanis KK: Neurocognitive deficit in schizophrenia: a quantitative review of the evidence. Neuropsychology 12:426–445, 1998

Hoff AL, Shuka S, Aronson T, et al: Failure to differentiate bipolar disorder from schizophrenia on measures of neuropsychological function. Schizophr Res 3:253–260, 1990

Hoff AL, Riordan H, O'Donnell DW, et al: Cross-sectional and longitudinal neuropsychological test findings in first-episode schizophrenic patients. Schizophr Res 5:197–198, 1991

Hoff AL, Riordan H, O'Donnell DW, et al: Neuropsychological functioning of first-episode schizophreniform patients. Am J Psychiatry 49:898–903, 1992

Hoff AL, Sakuma M, Wieneke M, et al: Longitudinal follow-up study of patients with first-episode schizophrenia. Am J Psychiatry 156:1336–1341, 1999

Huttenlocher PR: Synaptic density in human frontal cortex-developmental changes and effects of aging. Brain Res 163:195–205, 1979

Imbibo BP, Troetel WM, Martelli P, et al: A 6-month, placebo-controlled trial of eptastigmine in Alzheimer's disease. Dement Geriatr Cogn Disord 11:17–24, 2000

Jacobsen LK, Rapoport JL: Research update: childhood-onset schizophrenia: implications of clinical and neurobehavioral research. J Child Psychol Psychiatry 39:101–113, 1998

Jaskiw GE, Juliano DM, Goldberg TE, et al: Cerebral ventricular enlargement in schizophreniform disorder does not progress: a seven-year follow-up study. Schizophr Res 14:23–28, 1994

Jernigan TL, Tallal P: Late changes in brain morphology observable with MRI. Devel Med Child Neurol 32:379–385, 1990

Jernigan T, Zisook S, Heaton RK, et al: Magnetic resonance imaging abnormalities in the lenticular nuclei and cerebral cortex in schizophrenia. Arch Gen Psychiatry 48:881–890, 1991

Johnstone EC, Owens DGC, Bydder OM, et al: The spectrum of structural brain changes in schizophrenia: age of onset as a predictor of cognitive and clinical impairments and their cerebral correlates. Psychol Med 19:91–103, 1989

Jones P: The early origins of schizophrenia. Br Med Bull 53:135–155, 1997

Jones P, Done DJ: From birth to onset: a developmental perspective of schizophrenia in two national birth cohorts, in Neurodevelopment and Adult Psychopathology. Edited by Keshaven MS, Murray RM. Cambridge, United Kingdom, Cambridge University Press, 1997, pp 119–136

Jones P, Murray RM: The genetics of schizophrenia is the genetics of neurodevelopment. Br J Psychiatry 158:615–623, 1991

Jones P, Rodgers B, Murray R, et al: Child developmental risk factors for adult schizophrenia in the British 1946 birth cohort. Lancet 344:1398–1402, 1994

Keefe RSE, Silva SG, Perkins DG, et al: The effects of atypical antipsychotic drugs on neurocognitive impairment in schizophrenia: a review and meta-analysis. Schizophr Bull 25:201–222, 1999

Kenny J, Meltzer HY: The role of attention in higher cortical functions in schizophrenia. J Neuropsychiatry Clin Neurosci 3:269–275, 1991

Kenny JT, Friedman L, Findling RL, et al: Cognitive impairment in adolescents with schizophrenia. Am J Psychiatry 154:1613–1615, 1997

Kern RS, Wallace CJ, Hellman SG, et al: A training procedure for remediating WCST deficits in chronic psychotic patients: an adaptation of errorless learning principles. J Psychiatr Res 30:283–294, 1996

Kern RS, Green MF, Marshall Jr BD, et al: Risperidone versus Haldol on secondary memory: can newer medications aid learning? Schizophr Bull 25:223–232, 1999

Keshaven MS, Anderson S, Pettegrew JW: Is schizophrenia due to excessive synaptic pruning in the prefrontal cortex? The Feinberg hypothesis revisited. J Psychiatry Res 28:239–265, 1994

Klonoff H, Fibiger CH, Hutton GH: Neuropsychological patterns in chronic schizophrenia. J Nerv Ment Dis 150:291–300, 1970

Kolakowska T, Williams AO, Ardern M, et al: Schizophrenia with good and poor outcome: early clinical features, responses to neuroleptics and signs of organic dysfunction. Br J Psychiatry 146:229–246, 1985

Kremen WS, Buka SL, Seidman LJ, et al: IQ decline during childhood and adult psychotic symptoms in a community sample: a 19-year longitudinal study. Am J Psychiatry 155:672–677, 1998

Lewis DA, Anderson SA, Rosenberg DR, et al: Postnatal refinements of prefrontal cortical circuitry and schizophrenia. Schizophr Res 15:29–30, 1995

Lezak MD: Neuropsychological Assessment, 2nd Edition. New York, Oxford University Press, 1983

Loranger AW: Sex differences in age at onset of schizophrenia. Arch Gen Psychiatry 41:157–161, 1984

Lubin A, Geiseking CG, Williams HL: Direct measurement of cognitive deficit in schizophrenia. J Consult Psychol 26:139–143, 1962

Martin JP, Friedmeyer MH, Sterne AL, et al: IQ deficit in schizophrenia: a test of competing theories. J Clin Psychol 33:667–672, 1977

McClellan JM, Werry JS, Ham M: A follow-up study of early onset psychosis: comparison between outcome diagnoses of schizophrenia, mood disorders, and personality disorders. J Autism Develop Dis 23:616–635, 1993

McKenna PJ, Lund CE, Mortimer AN: Negative symptoms: relationship to other schizophrenic symptom classes. Br J Psychiatry 155:104–107, 1989

Meltzer HY, McGurk SR: The effects of clozapine, risperidone, and olanzapine on cognitive function in schizophrenia. Schizophr Bull 25:233–255, 1999

Moran LJ, Gorham DR, Holtzman WH: Vocabulary knowledge and usage of schizophrenic subjects: a six-year follow-up. J Abnorm Soc Psychol 61:246–265, 1962

Morice R: Cognitive inflexibility and prefrontal dysfunction in schizophrenia and mania. Br J Psychiatry 157:50–54, 1990

Murray RM, Lewis SW, Owen MJ, et al: The neurodevelopmental origins of dementia Praecox, in Schizophrenia: The Major Issues. Edited by Bebbington P, McGuffen P. London, England, William Heinman, 1988, pp 90–107

Nuechterlein LH, Dawson ME: Information processing and attentional functioning in the developmental course of schizophrenic disorders. Schizophr Bull 10:160–203, 1984

O'Carroll RE, Russell HH, Lawrie SM, et al: Errorless learning and the cognitive rehabilitation of memory-impaired schizophrenic patients. Psychol Med 29:105–112, 1999

Perry E, Walker M, Grace J, et al: Acetylcholine in mind: a neurotransmitter correlate of consciousness? Trends Neurosci 22:273–280, 1999

Purdon SE: Measuring neuropsychological change in schizophrenia with novel antipsychotic medications. J Psychiatry Neurosci 25:108–116, 2000

Purdon SE, Jones BD, Stip E, et al: Neuropsychological change in early phase schizophrenia during 12 months of treatment with olanzapine, risperidone, or haloperidol: the Canadian Collaborative Group for research in schizophrenia. Arch Gen Psychiatry 57:249–258, 2000

Purohit DP, Davidson M, Perl DP, et al: Severe cognitive impairment in elderly schizophrenic patients: a clinicopathological study. Biol Psychiatry 33:255–260, 1993

Randolph C, Goldberg TE, Weinberger DR: The neuropsychology of schizophrenia, in Clinical Neuropsychology. Edited by Heilman KM, Valenstein E. New York, Oxford University Press, 1993, pp 499–522

Ruff RM, Niemann H, Troster AI, et al: Effectiveness of behavioral management in rehabilitation, in Neurobehavioral Sequelae of Traumatic Brain Injury. Edited by Woods RLI. New York, Taylor & Francis, 1993, pp 305–334

Rund BR, Landro NI: Memory in schizophrenia and affective disorder. Scand J Psychol 36:37–46, 1995

Russell AJ, Munro JC, Jones P, et al: Schizophrenia and the myth of intellectual decline. Am J Psychiatry 154:635–639, 1997

Saykin AJ, Gur RC, Gur RE, et al: Neuropsychological function in schizophrenia: selective impairment in memory and learning. Arch Gen Psychiatry 48:618–624, 1991

Saykin AJ, Shtasel DL, Gur RE, et al: Neuropsychological deficits in neuroleptic naïve patients with first-episode schizophrenia. Arch Gen Psychiatry 51:124–131, 1994

Schulz SC, Koller MM, Kishore PR, et al: Ventricular enlargement in teenage patients with schizophrenia spectrum disorder. Am J Psychiatry 140:1592–1595, 1983

Schneider SG, Asarnow RF: A comparison between the cognitive/neuropsychological impairment of non-retarded autistic and schizophrenic children. J Abnorm Child Psychol 15:29–46, 1987

Schwartzman AE, Douglas VI: Intellectual loss in schizophrenia: part I. Can J Psychol 16:1–10, 1962

Schwartzman AE, Douglas VI, Muir WF: Intellectual loss in schizophrenia: part II. Can J Psychol 16:161–168, 1962

Silverstein ML, Harrow M, Bryson GJ: Neuropsychological prognosis and clinical recovery. Psychiatry Res 52:265–272, 1994

Small IF, Small JG, Millstein V, et al: Neuropsychological observations with psychosis and somatic treatment: neuropsychological examination of psychiatric patients. J Nerv Ment Dis 155:6–13, 1972

Sohlberg MM, White O, Evans E, et al: Background and initial case studies of the effects of prospective memory training. Brain Injury 6:129–138, 1992

Strauss ME, Prescott CA, Gutterman DF, et al: Span of apprehension deficits in schizophrenia and mania. Schizophr Bull 13:699–704, 1987

Tamlyn A, McKenna PJ, Mortimer AM, et al: Memory impairment in schizophrenia: its extant, affiliations and neuropsychological character. Psychiatry Med 22:1–15, 1992

Turner SW, Toone BK, Brett-Jones JR: Computerized tomography scan changes in early schizophrenia-preliminary findings. Psychol Med 16:219–225, 1986

van Os J, Jones P, Lewis GH, et al: Evidence for similar developmental precursors of chronic affective illness and schizophrenia in a general population birth cohort. Arch Gen Psychiatry 54:625–631, 1997

Velligan DI, Mahurin RK, Diamond PL, et al: The functional significance of symptomatology and cognitive function in schizophrenics. Schizophr Res 25:21–31, 1997

Weinberger D: Implications of normal brain development for the pathogenesis of schizophrenia. Arch Gen Psychiatry 44:660–669, 1987

Weinberger DR, Berman KF, Suddath R, et al: Evidence of dysfunction of prefrontal-limbic network in schizophrenia: a magnetic resonance imaging and cerebral blood flow study of discordant monozygotic twins. Am J Psychiatry 149:890–897, 1992

Wilson BA, Moffat N: Clinical Management of Memory Problems, 2nd Edition. London, Chapman & Hall, 1992

Wykes T, Reeder C, Corner J, et al: The effects of neurocognitive remediation on executive processing in patients with schizophrenia. Schizophr Bull 25:291–307, 1999

Afterword

S. Charles Schulz, M.D.
Robert B. Zipursky, M.D.

In concluding this volume on the early stages of schizophrenia, we thought it important to summarize and integrate the findings of the contributors. We begin with a brief summary of the recent data on the early stages of schizophrenia presented in the preceding chapters. We then provide suggestions for an optimal clinical approach to patients in the early stages of schizophrenia or related psychotic illness, and conclude by highlighting points for an integrated approach to young people recently diagnosed with schizophrenia.

What Have We Learned Recently?

Perhaps the most important lesson that the field has learned from studying patients in their first episode of schizophrenia is that of hope. Results of the Hillside Hospital study described in this volume indicate that approximately three out of four patients have a full remission from their first episode. In addition, case series studies in adolescents show new medicines to be well tolerated and effective early in the illness. We are hopeful that outcomes will continue to improve with the use of specific psychosocial interventions along with pharmacologic innovations.

The symptoms of schizophrenia are similar, whether one is working with adults, adolescents, or even children in their first episode. The diagnosis of schizophrenia can be made through clinical interviewing with patients, families, and other informants. It is particularly important in the early stages of psychosis to identify any medical causes of psychosis and to give careful consideration to the possibility that depression or mania might better explain the clinical presentation.

The field of psychiatry has been appropriately concerned about the stability of psychiatric diagnosis in the early stages of illness. A cautious approach was clearly warranted when pharmacologic interventions carried substantial side effects, including a high risk of tardive dyskinesia. In some cases, there may also be substantial diagnostic uncertainty in the early years of the illness. The enormous stigma that has been associated with the diagnosis of schizophrenia has also contributed to the reluctance to make the diagnosis early in the course of illness. However, recent first-episode and early-stage studies, as described in the Chapter 2 by Bromet and colleagues, show that the diagnosis of schizophrenia made at baseline has substantial stability over time. If the diagnosis can be made with confidence, if effective medications can be prescribed that are well tolerated and safe, and if reducing the length of untreated psychosis can improve long-term outcome, then a highly compelling argument can be made for early intervention.

Is it possible that intervening early in the illness may affect the underlying neurobiology of schizophrenia? Ultimately, this depends on whether the neuropathological basis of schizophrenia is present from early in life and remains static over time or whether it is progressive over some phase of the illness. Although much evidence suggests that the brain abnormalities reported in patients with schizophrenia are present before the onset of illness, the recent studies at the National Institute of Mental Health on teenagers with childhood-onset illness (described in Chapter 7 by Kumra and colleagues) suggest that there may be a limited progressive component to these brain abnormalities. If there is an active disease occurring in the brain in the early stages of the illness, it is conceivable that new therapies could be developed that would limit this process.

Not only do patients with childhood- and adolescence-onset schizophrenia have abnormalities on computed tomography and magnetic resonance imaging scans that are similar to those with adult-onset forms of the illness, but they also demonstrate similar difficulties in cognitive functioning, as assessed by formal neuropsychological testing. The cognitive difficulties noted by Kenny and Friedman in Chapter 9 are present even in patients who are ambulatory and essentially in remission. It is important to establish whether these deficits antedate the onset of illness or, alternatively, develop early in the course of the illness. This knowledge will help inform us about whether the most appropriate strategies for approaching these difficulties early in the illness will involve prevention or rehabilitation.

In the area of psychopharmacologic treatment of patients in the early stages of schizophrenia, first-episode studies of young adults have shown some interesting responses to very divergent protocols. For example, Lieberman and colleagues (see Chapter 3), following a traditional medication protocol, have found a very high remission rate for patients followed for the first year of their illness. This is an encouraging result and a cause for optimism in approaching younger patients. Using a markedly different pharmacologic approach, Zipursky and colleagues (see Chapter 4) at the University of Toronto have described success with much lower doses of traditional antipsychotic medications. Their more tailored approach to pharmacological management takes place in a specialized milieu with staff dedicated full time to the treatment of first-episode patients. What is becoming increasingly clear is that a large majority of first-episode patients have excellent responses to treatment and that there are ways to facilitate these responses without substantial side effects, whether one is using atypical antipsychotic agents or low doses of typical agents. Much less evidence is available on the psychopharmacology of childhood- and adolescent-onset schizophrenia, but there is an emerging consensus that both typical and atypical antipsychotic medications are clearly effective for these patients. Although many patients respond well to initial treatment, it must be kept in mind that many young patients still respond poorly. Whether one is working with children, adolescents, or adults, there is good reason to believe that these patients may benefit from clozapine; it will likely be in their best interest to move to clozapine sooner rather than later.

The Overall Approach

The sciences of epidemiology, brain imaging, neuropsychology, and psychopharmacology are all promising tools for the exploration of the early stages of schizophrenia. The summary of recently accumulated information noted here provides a platform for a rational approach to young patients. However, clinical practice is more complex than the sum of the scientific findings. A major rationale for this book has been to introduce readers to important differences that arise in approaching the clinical care of patients in the early stages of the illness. Among the most striking differences are the needs and reactions of patients and their families early in the course of schizophrenia.

It is very important for clinicians to understand the profound feelings of stigma, depression, and loss of self-esteem experienced in the early stages of psychosis. As McCay and Ryan describe in Chapter 5, young people struggling with a first episode of psychosis need to be emotionally engaged in the treatment process. Developing an empathic approach to young people at this early stage of this illness can go a long way in helping them to overcome the challenge of recovering from a first psychotic episode. The individual and group approaches that best meet the needs of these patients likely differ substantially from the approaches used for patients at later stages of schizophrenia. Similarly, as Collins has pointed out in Chapter 6, approaches developed for working with the families of adult patients with severe and persistent forms of schizophrenia are not likely to be transferable to young families with teens or young adults in the early stages of schizophrenia. Davies, as described in the chapter on adolescent schizophrenia, has studied the responses of young families to a group of psychiatric illnesses and found a variety of coping and response patterns that are important to consider in treatment planning. Helping patients and families cope with a first episode of psychosis remains among our greatest clinical challenges. If it were possible to prevent the development of the first episode of acute psychosis, as McGorry and his colleagues suggest in Chapter 1, patients and families might be spared much of the trauma and suffering that they now experience.

An Integrated Approach

It is recognized that not every setting may be able to replicate the specialized programs that have been established for first-episode patients in Toronto, Canada; on Long Island, New York; and in Melbourne, Australia. However, wherever one works, recognition of the major issues involved in diagnosis, early course of illness, psychopharmacology, and psychosocial management of individuals and families is important for ensuring the best possible outcomes. We believe that some of the major factors useful for an integrated approach to patients in the early stage of schizophrenia are:

• Individuals who present in the early phase of psychosis require careful clinical diagnostic evaluation, especially for medical illnesses, drug use, and mood disorders. At the same time, an understanding of the impact of psychosis on the individual needs to be appreciated.

• Families need to be engaged as soon as possible in the treatment process. The emotional and educational needs of each family must be assessed so services can be provided that fit their specific needs and capacity to participate.

- Antipsychotic medications should be initiated promptly while patients are still early in their clinical course. Medications should be prescribed in a way that minimizes side effects and maximizes long-term compliance. This usually involves treatment with atypical antipsychotic medication or low doses of typical antipsychotic medications. Clozapine should be considered early on in the face of poor response to treatment, whether one is working with children, teenagers, or adults in their first episode.

- Maintenance of remission involves a number of these interventions woven together. We believe that the best outcomes can be achieved by using a combination of maintenance medication; individual and group psychotherapies for young people; appropriately designed individual or multifamily group interventions; and strategies designed to address the individual's difficulties in vocational, educational, and social functioning.

The studies and experiences described in this book address a crucial stage of schizophrenia. We believe that early recognition, an assertive therapeutic approach, and continued integrated multidisciplinary treatment strategies are important for optimizing the overall outcome of these young patients and their families.

Index

Page numbers printed in **boldface** type refer to tables or figures.